Translational Research in Audiology

Translational Research in Audiology

Editor

Agnieszka Szczepek

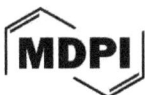

Basel • Beijing • Wuhan • Barcelona • Belgrade • Novi Sad • Cluj • Manchester

Editor
Agnieszka Szczepek
ORL, Head and Neck Surgery
Charité – Universitätsmedizin
Berlin
Berlin
Germany

Editorial Office
MDPI
St. Alban-Anlage 66
4052 Basel, Switzerland

This is a reprint of articles from the Special Issue published online in the open access journal *Audiology Research* (ISSN 2039-4349) (available at: www.mdpi.com/journal/audiolres/special_issues/translational_research_audiology).

For citation purposes, cite each article independently as indicated on the article page online and as indicated below:

Lastname, A.A.; Lastname, B.B. Article Title. *Journal Name* **Year**, *Volume Number*, Page Range.

ISBN 978-3-0365-9161-2 (Hbk)
ISBN 978-3-0365-9160-5 (PDF)
doi.org/10.3390/books978-3-0365-9160-5

© 2023 by the authors. Articles in this book are Open Access and distributed under the Creative Commons Attribution (CC BY) license. The book as a whole is distributed by MDPI under the terms and conditions of the Creative Commons Attribution-NonCommercial-NoDerivs (CC BY-NC-ND) license.

Contents

About the Editor vii

Preface ix

Agnieszka J. Szczepek
Translational Research in Audiology
Reprinted from: *Audiol. Res.* **2023**, *13*, 721-723, doi:10.3390/audiolres13050063 1

Agnieszka J. Szczepek, Ewa Domarecka and Heidi Olze
Translational Research in Audiology: Presence in the Literature
Reprinted from: *Audiol. Res.* **2022**, *12*, 674-679, doi:10.3390/audiolres12060064 4

Ewa Domarecka and Agnieszka J. Szczepek
Universal Recommendations on Planning and Performing the Auditory Brainstem Responses (ABR) with a Focus on Mice and Rats
Reprinted from: *Audiol. Res.* **2023**, *13*, 441-458, doi:10.3390/audiolres13030039 10

Cristina Maria Blebea, Violeta Necula, Monica Potara, Maximilian George Dindelegan, Laszlo Peter Ujvary and Emil Claudiu Botan et al.
The Effect of Pluronic-Coated Gold Nanoparticles in Hearing Preservation Following Cochlear Implantation-Pilot Study
Reprinted from: *Audiol. Res.* **2022**, *12*, 466-475, doi:10.3390/audiolres12050047 28

Gusta van Zwieten, Jana V. P. Devos, Sonja A. Kotz, Linda Ackermans, Pia Brinkmann and Lobke Dauven et al.
A Protocol to Investigate Deep Brain Stimulation for Refractory Tinnitus: From Rat Model to the Set-Up of a Human Pilot Study
Reprinted from: *Audiol. Res.* **2022**, *13*, 49-63, doi:10.3390/audiolres13010005 38

Marc Fagelson
Tinnitus Education for Audiologists Is a Ship at Sea: Is It Coming or Going?
Reprinted from: *Audiol. Res.* **2023**, *13*, 389-397, doi:10.3390/audiolres13030034 53

Aleksandra Bendowska, Roksana Malak, Agnieszka Zok and Ewa Baum
The Ethics of Translational Audiology
Reprinted from: *Audiol. Res.* **2022**, *12*, 273-280, doi:10.3390/audiolres12030028 62

Raul Sanchez-Lopez, Mengfan Wu, Michal Fereczkowski, Sébastien Santurette, Monika Baumann and Borys Kowalewski et al.
Towards Auditory Profile-Based Hearing-Aid Fittings: BEAR Rationale and Clinical Implementation
Reprinted from: *Audiol. Res.* **2022**, *12*, 564-573, doi:10.3390/audiolres12050055 70

Ryota Shimokura
Sound Quality Factors Inducing the Autonomous Sensory Meridian Response
Reprinted from: *Audiol. Res.* **2022**, *12*, 574-584, doi:10.3390/audiolres12050056 80

Mohamed Bassiouni, Sophia Marie Häußler, Stefan Gräbel, Agnieszka J. Szczepek and Heidi Olze
Lateralization Pattern of the Weber Tuning Fork Test in Longstanding Unilateral Profound Hearing Loss: Implications for Cochlear Implantation
Reprinted from: *Audiol. Res.* **2022**, *12*, 347-356, doi:10.3390/audiolres12040036 91

Dominik Péus, Shaumiya Sellathurai, Nicolas Newcomb, Kurt Tschopp and Andreas Radeloff
The Otoprotective Effect of Ear Cryotherapy: Systematic Review and Future Perspectives
Reprinted from: *Audiol. Res.* **2022**, *12*, 377-387, doi:10.3390/audiolres12040038 . . . . **101**

Don McFerran and Laurence McKenna
In Memoriam: David Mark Baguley
Reprinted from: *Audiol. Res.* **2022**, *12*, 585-588, doi:10.3390/audiolres12060057 . . . . **112**

About the Editor

Agnieszka Szczepek

Agnieszka J. Szczepek received an M.Sc. in Microbiology/Immunology (University of Warsaw, Warsaw, Poland, 1986) and a Ph.D. in Medical Sciences (University of Alberta, Edmonton, AB, Canada, 1999). She returned to Europe in 2000 at the invitation of the Max Planck Society to work at the Institute of Infection Biology in Berlin, Germany. In 2006, she joined the Department of Otolaryngology, Head, and Neck Surgery at Charité-Universitätsmedizin Berlin, Germany, as a researcher and academic teacher. Since then, her research has focused on clinical and experimental audiology, otology, and laryngology. Since 2017, she has also taught at the Collegium Medicum in Zielona Góra, Poland.

Preface

The idea of publishing a collection of articles on translational audiology has been with me for a long time. During my Ph.D. studies at the University of Alberta in Edmonton, Canada, I followed the then-much-promoted translational approach. After transitioning to hearing research, I noticed that the translational approach was not prominent in the discipline. This lack of visibility is not due to a lack of relevant research but to the fact that the term "translational audiology" is extremely rarely used.

The collection of articles contained in this reprint was created to change this state of affairs and to stimulate the interest of others working in the field of experimental or clinical audiology. It is my hope that translational audiology will gain attention as a scientific discipline and that we will see much more research in this area.

The publication of this reprint was made possible thanks to all the authors and research groups who contributed to it. A big thank you! Second, but no less important, are our families and loved ones who have patiently endured our work on weekends, holidays, and late nights. Third, and perhaps most important, are the patients who have contributed directly by participating in the studies or indirectly by consenting to using their clinical data and asking questions that stimulate translational audiology research.

This work is dedicated to the memory of Prof. Rev. David Baguley, one of the finest audiologists I have ever known.

Agnieszka Szczepek
Editor

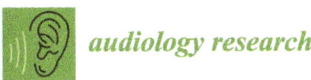

Editorial

Translational Research in Audiology

Agnieszka J. Szczepek [1,2]

1 Department of Otorhinolaryngology, Head and Neck Surgery, Charité-Universitätsmedizin Berlin, Corporate Member of Freie Universität Berlin, Humboldt-Universität zu Berlin, 10117 Berlin, Germany; agnes.szczepek@charite.de
2 Faculty of Medicine and Health Sciences, University of Zielona Gora, 65-046 Zielona Gora, Poland

The importance of translational research in the medical sciences is growing logarithmically, as this type of research provides the translation of basic research into a clinical product (a drug, therapeutic agent or means of monitoring a disease), as well as the inverse translation of clinical findings into basic research models. This special issue is devoted to translational research in audiology. Unfortunately, the terms "translational audiology" or "translational research in audiology" are still rarely used which encourages a change to increase the visibility of such publications. Among the many benefits associated with using the term "translational audiology" is identifying this type of research as a distinct stream in the science of audiology and emphasizing its practical application in clinical work. How often the term "translational audiology" is used in the literature, what articles have been published using the term, and the rationale and implications of such publications can be found in the review "Translational Research in Audiology: Presence in the Literature" [1].

The translational process often begins in the basic research laboratory. It is essential for clinical success that basic research experiments are reproducible. One of the manuscripts in our special issue addresses this by providing recommendations for performing auditory brainstem response (ABR) in small animals. These recommendations developed by Domarecka et al. are intended to improve the reproducibility of basic audiological research ("Universal Recommendations on Planning and Performing the Auditory Brainstem Responses (ABR) with a Focus on Mice and Rats") [2].

ABR was the audiometric method used by Blebea et al. to measure the hearing thresholds of rats following mechanical injury to the cochlea when one ear was treated with Pluronic-coated gold nanoparticles containing dexamethasone and the other ear was treated with dexamethasone alone. The comparative analysis of the ABR results demonstrated the benefit of using Pluronic-coated gold nanoparticles over dexamethasone alone ("The Effect of Pluronic-Coated Gold Nanoparticles in Hearing Preservation Following Cochlear Implantation—Pilot Study") [3]. The investigators suggested that the results of this study could be translated to modify the methods of cochlear implantation in patients with residual hearing, such as those with Meniere's disease.

A classic example of the translational approach in audiology was proposed by van Zwieten et al. in a paper suggesting the use of deep brain stimulation to treat refractory tinnitus ("A Protocol for Deep Brain Stimulation for Refractory Tinnitus: From Rat Model to Human Pilot Study") [4]. The health problems associated with tinnitus (e.g., insomnia or difficulty concentrating) can sometimes be extremely distressing, prompting patients and researchers to seek unusual solutions. In order to implement such a solution, the authors developed a translational protocol based on the results of the animal studies.

Tinnitus therapy is the responsibility of many medical disciplines, and many patients seeking help turn to audiologists. However, the education of audiologists varies from country to country and sometimes from one school of audiology to another. In addition, the job title "audiologist" may have various meanings in different settings. This is associated with diverse levels of responsibility and professional obligations. In a communication paper,

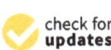

Citation: Szczepek, A.J. Translational Research in Audiology. *Audiol. Res.* 2023, 13, 721–723. https://doi.org/10.3390/audiolres13050063

Received: 18 September 2023
Accepted: 21 September 2023
Published: 25 September 2023

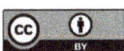

Copyright: © 2023 by the author. Licensee MDPI, Basel, Switzerland. This article is an open access article distributed under the terms and conditions of the Creative Commons Attribution (CC BY) license (https://creativecommons.org/licenses/by/4.0/).

Marc Fagelson discusses tinnitus-related training for audiologists in the USA ("Tinnitus education for audiologists is a ship at sea: is it coming or going?") [5].

Implantable hearing aids have changed the lives of many people who have lost their hearing or were born deaf. However, regardless of the effectiveness of the treatment, implantation should not be applied when people are unwilling to be treated or in minors if their guardians do not consent. This issue and related reasons are further discussed by Bendowska et al. in the article "The Ethics of Translational Audiology" which raises awareness about treating the deaf community with dignity and respecting their wishes, which are sometimes at odds with those of hearing people [6].

Sanchez-Lopez et al. provided an excellent example of translational research that focused on translating a hearing aid fitting strategy to the setting needed for large clinical trials ("Towards auditory profile-based hearing-aid fittings: BEAR rationale and clinical implementation"). This group found the first fitting strategy that prescribes gain targets and adjusts advanced hearing aid features for the purpose of clinical research. Other applications could also benefit from using such a fitting strategy [7].

Ryota Shimokura tackled a very interesting subject of autonomous sensory meridian response (ASMR). ASMR is a tingling sensation originating on the scalp and progressing down the spine. Various sound or visual triggers can induce ASMR, and the manuscript "Sound Quality Factors Inducing the Autonomous Sensory Meridian Response" focused on characterizing sound that induces ASMR [8]. The interesting finding of that study was that the human voice could trigger stronger ASMR than the sounds of nature.

The paper by Bassiouni et al., "Lateralization Pattern of the Weber Tuning Fork Test in Longstanding Unilateral Profound Hearing Loss: Implications for Cochlear Implantation" is thought-provoking [9]. It shows that a significant proportion of patients with unilateral hearing loss, despite the unilateral hearing commonly associated with Weber test lateralization, report a lack of such lateralization. Bassiouni suggests that since the duration of deafness correlates positively with this unexpected effect, the loss of Weber lateralization in unilateral deaf patients may result from a central adaptation of sound processing pathway. This finding needs to be considered in cochlear implant candidates. The authors also postulate the need for reverse translational research in this area.

A very interesting topic of the therapeutic implication of low temperature on the outcome of inner ear diseases was put on the spot in a literature review paper, "The Otoprotective Effect of Ear Cryotherapy: Systematic Review and Future Perspectives" [10]. However, the basic research models used whole-body cooling techniques and could not be translated to clinical settings. The general conclusion of the review authors was that the therapeutic use of low temperatures is a promising approach and should be explored further.

There were dark clouds on the horizon in June 2022 when we received the sad news of the untimely and unexpected death of our long-time colleague and wonderful human being—Rev. Prof. David Baguley. David Baguley was active in translational audiology and contributed many publications and chapters to a book on the subject. Don McFerran (ENT surgeon) and Laurence McKenna (clinical psychologist) knew David very well and have taken on the challenge of describing the outline of his life and achievements as a fulfilled audiologist, a beloved Church of England clergyman, an admired academic mentor and, above all, a trusted friend, colleague and family man ("In Memoriam: David Mark Baguley") [11].

I would like to dedicate this special issue to the memory of Rev. Prof. David Mark Baguley.

Conflicts of Interest: The author declares no conflict of interest.

References

1. Szczepek, A.J.; Domarecka, E.; Olze, H. Translational Research in Audiology: Presence in the Literature. *Audiol. Res.* **2022**, *12*, 674–679. [CrossRef]
2. Domarecka, E.; Szczepek, A.J. Universal Recommendations on Planning and Performing the Auditory Brainstem Responses (ABR) with a Focus on Mice and Rats. *Audiol. Res.* **2023**, *13*, 441–458. [CrossRef]

3. Blebea, C.M.; Necula, V.; Potara, M.; Dindelegan, M.G.; Ujvary, L.P.; Botan, E.C.; Maniu, A.A.; Cosgarea, M. The Effect of Pluronic-Coated Gold Nanoparticles in Hearing Preservation Following Cochlear Implantation-Pilot Study. *Audiol. Res.* **2022**, *12*, 466–475. [CrossRef] [PubMed]
4. van Zwieten, G.; Devos, J.V.P.; Kotz, S.A.; Ackermans, L.; Brinkmann, P.; Dauven, L.; George, E.L.J.; Janssen, A.M.L.; Kremer, B.; Leue, C.; et al. A Protocol to Investigate Deep Brain Stimulation for Refractory Tinnitus: From Rat Model to the Set-Up of a Human Pilot Study. *Audiol. Res.* **2023**, *13*, 49–63. [CrossRef] [PubMed]
5. Fagelson, M. Tinnitus Education for Audiologists Is a Ship at Sea: Is It Coming or Going? *Audiol. Res.* **2023**, *13*, 389–397. [CrossRef] [PubMed]
6. Bendowska, A.; Malak, R.; Zok, A.; Baum, E. The Ethics of Translational Audiology. *Audiol. Res.* **2022**, *12*, 273–280. [CrossRef] [PubMed]
7. Sanchez-Lopez, R.; Wu, M.; Fereczkowski, M.; Santurette, S.; Baumann, M.; Kowalewski, B.; Piechowiak, T.; Bisgaard, N.; Ravn, G.; Narayanan, S.K.; et al. Towards Auditory Profile-Based Hearing-Aid Fittings: BEAR Rationale and Clinical Implementation. *Audiol. Res.* **2022**, *12*, 564–573. [CrossRef] [PubMed]
8. Shimokura, R. Sound Quality Factors Inducing the Autonomous Sensory Meridian Response. *Audiol. Res.* **2022**, *12*, 574–584. [CrossRef] [PubMed]
9. Bassiouni, M.; Häußler, S.M.; Gräbel, S.; Szczepek, A.J.; Olze, H. Lateralization Pattern of the Weber Tuning Fork Test in Longstanding Unilateral Profound Hearing Loss: Implications for Cochlear Implantation. *Audiol. Res.* **2022**, *12*, 347–356. [CrossRef] [PubMed]
10. Péus, D.; Sellathurai, S.; Newcomb, N.; Tschopp, K.; Radeloff, A. The Otoprotective Effect of Ear Cryotherapy: Systematic Review and Future Perspectives. *Audiol. Res.* **2022**, *12*, 377–387. [CrossRef] [PubMed]
11. McFerran, D.; McKenna, L. In Memoriam: David Mark Baguley. *Audiol. Res.* **2022**, *12*, 585–588. [CrossRef] [PubMed]

Disclaimer/Publisher's Note: The statements, opinions and data contained in all publications are solely those of the individual author(s) and contributor(s) and not of MDPI and/or the editor(s). MDPI and/or the editor(s) disclaim responsibility for any injury to people or property resulting from any ideas, methods, instructions or products referred to in the content.

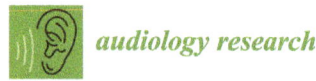

Review

Translational Research in Audiology: Presence in the Literature

Agnieszka J. Szczepek [1,2,*], Ewa Domarecka [1] and Heidi Olze [1]

1. Department of Otorhinolaryngology, Head and Neck Surgery, Charité–Universitätsmedizin Berlin, 10117 Berlin, Germany
2. Faculty of Medicine and Health Sciences, University of Zielona Gora, 65-046 Zielona Gora, Poland
* Correspondence: agnes.szczepek@charite.de

Abstract: Translational research is a process that focuses on advancing basic research-based clinical solutions and is characterized by a structured process accelerating the implementation of scientific discoveries in healthcare. Translational research originated in oncology but has spread to other disciplines in recent decades. A translational project may refer to pharmacological research, the development of non-pharmacological therapies, or to disease monitoring processes. Its stages are divided into basic research focused on the clinical problem (T0), testing the developed means in humans (T1), conducting trials with patients (T2), implementation and dissemination of successful approaches (T3), and improving community health (T4). Many audiological studies are translational in nature. Accordingly, this scoping review aimed to evaluate the use of the terms "translational audiology" and "translational research in audiology" in the literature and examine the goals of the identified studies. PubMed and Web of Science search identified only two publications meeting the search criteria. We conclude that identifying translational audiological studies in the literature may be hampered by the lack of use of the terms "translational audiology" or "translational research". We suggest using these terms when describing translational work in audiology, with a view to facilitating the identification of this type of research and credit it appropriately.

Keywords: audiology; translational research; translational science; translational audiology

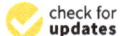

Citation: Szczepek, A.J.; Domarecka, E.; Olze, H. Translational Research in Audiology: Presence in the Literature. *Audiol. Res.* 2022, 12, 674–679. https://doi.org/10.3390/audiolres12060064

Academic Editor: Andrea Ciorba

Received: 21 October 2022
Accepted: 25 November 2022
Published: 28 November 2022

Publisher's Note: MDPI stays neutral with regard to jurisdictional claims in published maps and institutional affiliations.

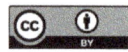

Copyright: © 2022 by the authors. Licensee MDPI, Basel, Switzerland. This article is an open access article distributed under the terms and conditions of the Creative Commons Attribution (CC BY) license (https://creativecommons.org/licenses/by/4.0/).

1. Introduction

Translational research (TR) is a biomedical investigation focusing on developing, implementing, and disseminating clinical therapeutic means, and its approach is a well-defined process involving "bench-to-bedside" laboratory investigations aiming to develop therapeutic means (T1), clinical trials that use the developed means (T2), implementation and dissemination of successful therapeutic strategy (T3), and studies of outcomes (T4) [1,2]. Additionally, "reverse translation" may be used to study observations made in the clinics during T2, using the "bedside-to-bench" approach (Figure 1) [3]. TR is a rapidly progressing discipline first introduced in oncology and spreading to all other biomedical specialties [4], including audiology [5].

Identifying research as "translational" helps others quickly recognize the study's aims and is critical for preparing grant proposals, developing new studies, or extracting data for systematic reviews or meta-analyses. Additionally, the term "translational audiology" creates a niche in biomedical disciplines and indicates a commitment to convert audiology-related basic findings into clinical approaches, thereby eventually improving the community's health. An efficient method to identify focused research is Medical Subject Heading (MeSH). MeSH is a stratified vocabulary created and provided by the National Library of Medicine and is used to describe the content of journal articles. Carrying out a search according to the subject content of journal articles rather than to the occurrence of a word or phrase [6] is particularly useful when gaining an understanding of the scope of a field.

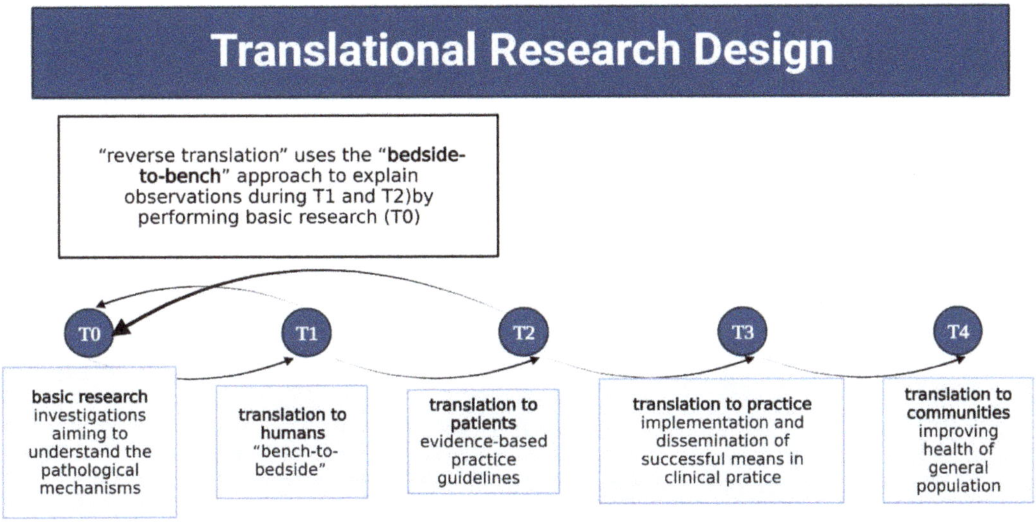

Figure 1. Types of translational research based on the description by Wichman et al. (2021) [2]. Created with BioRender.com.

Due to the anatomical and biological properties of the inner ear and the auditory pathways, progress in audiology can be achieved by solving clinical problems in clinical [7] or laboratory settings [8], software-simulated situations [9], animal models [10], or explanted tissues [11]. Numerous studies in audiology have a translational character, including research on preventing ototoxicity, EEG-based auditory tests (auditory brainstem responses, ABRs) of noise-exposed animals treated with protective substances, or development of tinnitus- or vertigo-related apps. However, the terms "translational audiology" or "translational research in audiology" seem to be rarely used to label such studies or publications. Hence, our research question was: *'Can translational research in audiology be identified in the literature based on the use of the phrase "translational audiology" or "translational research in audiology?"'*. Consequently, this scoping review aimed to map translational research in audiology indicated by MeSH terms in the scientific literature, to characterize the primary research goals in the identified research, and recommend future directions.

2. Materials and Methods

The search was performed in October 2022 using EndNote 20 without time window restrictions. Two databases (PubMed and Web of Science) were searched using Medical Subject Heading MeSH Terms (Pubmed) and title/keyword/abstract (Web of Science). The keywords used were: "translational audiology"; "translational research" AND "audiology"; and "translational science" AND "audiology". Inclusion criteria were English as a publication language and primary research; exclusion criteria were review articles, editorials, overviews, and commentaries.

The search retrieved 32 publications (Figure 2). Examination of PubMed with MeSH Terms "translational research" AND MeSH Terms "audiology" returned 3 hits; MeSH Terms "translational research" AND MeSH Terms "audiology"—3 papers; MeSH Terms "translational audiology"—10 hits; and MeSH Terms "translational science" AND MeSH Terms "audiology"—3 hits: 19 publications in total. The search of Web of Science (keyword/title/abstract) using the keyword "translational audiology" retrieved 6 hits; "translational research" AND "audiology"—5 hits; and "translational science" AND "audiology"—2 hits: 13 publications in total. Of these 32 publications, 18 duplicates were identified and removed. Abstracts of the remaining 14 publications were manually screened, and five records were removed because their topics did not involve translational audiology research. The rest of the publications were assessed for eligibility, and seven did not match the inclusion criteria (editorials, reviews, opinions, or overview papers).

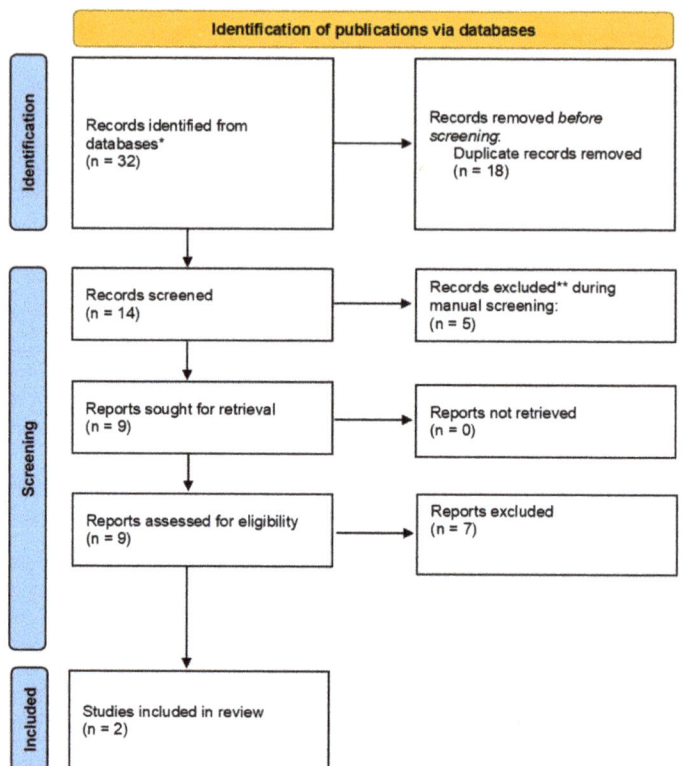

Figure 2. PRISMA flowchart visualizing the search and selection process. * Databases used: PubMed and Web of Science; ** reasons for exclusion: topic outside the scope of the review.

Two manuscripts were included in the detailed analysis, and the type of translational research used (T1–T4) and the main study aims were examined.

PubMed and the Web of Science are the most popular sources for publication searches. However, Google Scholar represents another essential search engine that screens not only the journals listed in PubMed or Web of Science but also books. To identify books published on the topic, we performed an additional search in Google Scholar using the terms "translational research" AND "audiology". That search retrieved 1790 hits; of them, 1220 were books, book chapters, or citations. A manual search identified three books that used the TR term and "audiology" in their titles (see Section 3.2).

3. Results
3.1. Journal Publications Identified in the Main Search

Two publications were included in this review for the data extraction [12,13]. The goal of the first publication (Kirk, K.I.; Prusick, L.; French, B.; Gotch, C.; Eisenberg, L.S.; Young, N. Assessing Spoken Word Recognition in Children Who Are Deaf or Hard of Hearing: A Translational Approach. Journal of the American Academy of Audiology 2012, 23, 464–475, doi:10.3766/jaaa.23.6.8.) was to "enhance our ability to estimate the real-world listening ability and to predict benefit from sensory aid use in children with varying degrees of hearing loss." The motivation behind that was a clinical observation that children with a cochlear implant performed poorly on word recognition tests despite their positive performance in real-life situations. That prompted the authors to return to the laboratories and redesign the word recognition tests. In translational research, such an approach represents T2 to T1 methodology (reverse translation). To achieve their goal, the authors have analyzed children's performance, identified the tests' shortcomings, and proposed solutions by introducing multimodal sentence tests optimized for children with CI (T3).

The second publication included in this review (Urquiza, R.; Lopez-Garcia, J. A new strategy for development of transducers for middle ear implants. Acta Oto-Laryngol 2015, 135, 135–139, doi:10.3109/00016489.2014.969381.) scrutinized the role of micro-electro-mechanical technology in the design and production of middle ear implants. The authors analyzed the technological and medical situations regarding the available expertise and product roadmap achievement related to T0, T1, and T2 translational steps.

3.2. Books Identified in the Additional Search

Using Google Scholar, we identified the following three books:

"Translational Research in Audiology, Neurotology, and the Hearing Sciences", with ten chapters discussing various aspects of translational research in the field [5].

"Translational Speech-Language Pathology and Audiology: Essays in Honor of Dr. Sadanand Singh", which contains information on translational research in general and then deals with the translational approach in audiology [14].

"Translational Perspectives in Auditory Neuroscience: Hearing Across the Life Span—Assessment and Disorders", which introduces the auditory system and discusses translational aspects of audiological diagnostics and therapies [15].

4. Discussion

At the beginning of this study, we asked the question: 'Can translational research in audiology be identified in the literature based on the use of the phrase "translational audiology" or "translational research in audiology?"'. The answer to this question is 'yes'; however, the MeSH term search identified only two peer-reviewed journal publications that met the inclusion criteria. The two manuscripts retrieved during the systematic search of journals had clearly defined translational character and specifically mentioned translational research in audiology. However, no stage of TR (T0–T4) was indicated in these papers and had to be deduced from the body of the text.

The results of the MeSH term search do not represent the actual volume of published translational research in audiology, which is substantially higher. Searches for a specific topic or term (without using TR as a keyword), such as creating or validating audiology-related questionnaires, developing therapeutic strategies for hearing loss, or anti-ototoxic strategies, retrieved hundreds of hits. That, in the light of our study, suggests that the researchers and clinicians are reluctant to use the term "translational audiology" or "translational research" in their published manuscripts. However, this was not the case regarding the books published in the recent decade [5,14,15]. Below, we attempt to analyze the possible reasons behind that reluctance and present incentives to use this terminology.

Translational research aims to implement research findings clinically and ensures that the new therapeutic or monitoring means will reach the appropriate community. The definition of translational research and the steps involved has evolved over the years. Therefore, the first reason for hesitating to use the term "translational research" in audiology could be the multiple meanings awarded to that term over time. These multiple meanings could have been induced by a constant revision of TR's definition [2,16] and a diverse perception of TR by different scientific fields, including for instance, viewing basic research as non-translational [17]. Supporting this view, in their analysis of publications from various medical disciplines, Krueger et al. showed that many scientific groups use the terminology "translational research" but understand it in various ways. [16]. No study so far has explored the understanding of the term TR among experimental or clinical audiologists.

The second reason behind the reluctant use of TR terminology in publications could be a lack of motivation. Calls for TR-targeted grants could enhance this motivation. For the past four years, the UK-based Royal National Institute for Deaf People and French Fondation Pour l'Audition have held a competition for research grants focused on translational research for hearing loss and tinnitus [18]. In the USA, the National Institute on Deafness and Other Communication Disorders (NIDCD) has offered this kind of grant for almost a decade. Nevertheless, securing a grant related to translational research makes TR more popular as a term but does not assure the use of it while publishing the research outcomes.

Apart from reluctance, the unfamiliarity of the audiological society with TR could also be a reason for the sparse use of that term in published work. Here, it would be suggested to propagate this term among the community of audiologists, for example, during scientific congresses or professional courses.

A final possible reason that could be responsible for the infrequent use of "translational audiology" may be the multidisciplinary approach often used in audiology research [19–21]. This approach can sometimes result in publishing with an emphasis on other disciplines, leaving translational audiology overshadowed by, e.g., neurology or otorhinolaryngology.

The obvious challenge is how to enhance the use of the term TR in audiology publications. One encouragement would be to emphasize that applying the term TR could increase the visibility of published studies. Recently, a bibliometric measure of translational science has been proposed to evaluate the translation of basic research into clinics [22]. This method tracks the practical implementation of preclinical research, resulting in the so-called translational score. While it is labor intensive, it focuses on the translational success of a specific manuscript and can also be used to track the practical success of steps T0–T4. An additional incentive would be the possibility of extending the scope of publishing to journals specializing in TR. Another effective solution to increase the popularity and use of the term TR could be an introduction of a well-defined subsection "Translational Audiology" or "Translational Research in Audiology" in specialized journals.

In conclusion, at present, identifying translational research in audiology using MeSH terms is challenging. It could be facilitated by adding TR to the keywords and methods section. Specifying particular translational steps (T0 to T4) could also aid in understanding the research design and lead to additional recognition and more significant credit in the field.

Author Contributions: Conceptualization, A.J.S.; methodology, A.J.S.; formal analysis, A.J.S. and E.D.; investigation, A.J.S. and E.D.; resources, H.O.; writing—original draft preparation, A.J.S.; writing—review and editing, A.J.S., E.D. and H.O.; visualization, A.J.S. All authors have read and agreed to the published version of the manuscript.

Funding: This research received no external funding.

Data Availability Statement: Not applicable.

Conflicts of Interest: The authors declare no conflict of interest.

References

1. Fort, D.G.; Herr, T.M.; Shaw, P.L.; Gutzman, K.E.; Starren, J.B. Mapping the evolving definitions of translational research. *Clin. Transl. Sci.* **2017**, *1*, 60–66. [CrossRef] [PubMed]
2. Wichman, C.; Smith, L.M.; Yu, F. A framework for clinical and translational research in the era of rigor and reproducibility. *Clin. Transl. Sci.* **2021**, *5*, e31. [CrossRef] [PubMed]
3. Shakhnovich, V. It's Time to Reverse our Thinking: The Reverse Translation Research Paradigm. *Clin. Transl. Sci.* **2018**, *11*, 98–99. [CrossRef] [PubMed]
4. Van der Laan, A.L.; Boenink, M. Beyond Bench and Bedside: Disentangling the Concept of Translational Research. *Health Care Anal.* **2015**, *23*, 32–49. [CrossRef] [PubMed]
5. Le Prell, C.G.; Lobarinas, E.; Popper, A.N.; Fay, R.R. *Translational Research in Audiology, Neurotology, and the Hearing Sciences*; Springer: Berlin/Heidelberg, Germany, 2016; Volume 58.
6. DeMars, M.M.; Perruso, C. MeSH and text-word search strategies: Precision, recall, and their implications for library instruction. *J. Med. Libr. Assoc.* **2022**, *110*, 23–33. [CrossRef] [PubMed]

7. Barrett, D.J.K.; Souto, D.; Pilling, M.; Baguley, D.M. An Exploratory Investigation of Pupillometry as a Measure of Tinnitus Intrusiveness on a Test of Auditory Short-Term Memory. *Ear Hear.* **2022**, *43*, 1540–1548. [CrossRef] [PubMed]
8. Searchfield, G.D.; Muñoz, D.J.; Thorne, P.R. Ensemble spontaneous activity in the guinea-pig cochlear nerve. *Hear. Res.* **2004**, *192*, 23–35. [CrossRef]
9. Buran, B.N.; McMillan, G.P.; Keshishzadeh, S.; Verhulst, S.; Bramhall, N.F. Predicting synapse counts in living humans by combining computational models with auditory physiology. *J. Acoust. Soc. Am.* **2022**, *151*, 561. [CrossRef] [PubMed]
10. Tserga, E.; Damberg, P.; Canlon, B.; Cederroth, C.R. Auditory synaptopathy in mice lacking the glutamate transporter GLAST and its impact on brain activity. *Prog. Brain Res.* **2021**, *262*, 245–261. [CrossRef] [PubMed]
11. Landegger, L.D.; Dilwali, S.; Stankovic, K.M. Neonatal Murine Cochlear Explant Technique as an In Vitro Screening Tool in Hearing Research. *J. Vis. Exp.* **2017**, *8*, 55704. [CrossRef]
12. Kirk, K.I.; Prusick, L.; French, B.; Gotch, C.; Eisenberg, L.S.; Young, N. Assessing Spoken Word Recognition in Children Who Are Deaf or Hard of Hearing: A Translational Approach. *J. Am. Acad. Audiol.* **2012**, *23*, 464–475. [CrossRef] [PubMed]
13. Urquiza, R.; Lopez-Garcia, J. A new strategy for development of transducers for middle ear implants. *Acta Oto-Laryngol.* **2015**, *135*, 135–139. [CrossRef] [PubMed]
14. Goldfarb, R. *Translational Speech-Language Pathology and Audiology: Essays in Honor of Dr. Sadanand Singh*; Plural Publishing: San Diego, CA, USA, 2012.
15. Tremblay, K.L.; Burkard, R.F. *Translational Perspectives in Auditory Neuroscience: Hearing Across the Life Span—Assessment and Disorders*; Plural Publishing: San Diego, CA, USA, 2012; Volume 2.
16. Krueger, A.K.; Hendriks, B.; Gauch, S. The multiple meanings of translational research in (bio)medical research. *Hist. Philos. Life Sci.* **2019**, *41*, 57. [CrossRef] [PubMed]
17. Flier, J.S.; Loscalzo, J. Categorizing biomedical research: The basics of translation. *FASEB J.* **2017**, *31*, 3210–3215. [CrossRef] [PubMed]
18. RNID. RNID-FPA Translational Grant. Available online: https://rnid.org.uk/hearing-research/im-a-researcher-looking-for-funding/translational-grant/ (accessed on 20 October 2022).
19. Hylton, J.B.; Leon-Salazar, V.; Anderson, G.C.; De Felippe, N.L. Multidisciplinary treatment approach in Treacher Collins syndrome. *J. Dent. Child.* **2012**, *79*, 15–21.
20. Simoes, J.P.; Daoud, E.; Shabbir, M.; Amanat, S.; Assouly, K.; Biswas, R.; Casolani, C.; Dode, A.; Enzler, F.; Jacquemin, L.; et al. Multidisciplinary Tinnitus Research: Challenges and Future Directions from the Perspective of Early Stage Researchers. *Front. Aging Neurosci.* **2021**, *13*, 647285. [CrossRef] [PubMed]
21. Cherney, L.R.; Gardner, P.; Logemann, J.A.; Newman, L.A.; O'Neil-Pirozzi, T.; Roth, C.R.; Solomon, N.P. The role of speech-language pathology and audiology in the optimal management of the service member returning from Iraq or Afghanistan with a blast-related head injury: Position of the Communication Sciences and Disorders Clinical Trials Research Group. *J. Head Trauma Rehabil.* **2010**, *25*, 219–224. [CrossRef] [PubMed]
22. Kim, Y.H.; Levine, A.D.; Nehl, E.J.; Walsh, J.P. A Bibliometric Measure of Translational Science. *Scientometrics* **2020**, *125*, 2349–2382. [CrossRef]

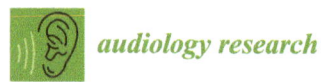

Article

Universal Recommendations on Planning and Performing the Auditory Brainstem Responses (ABR) with a Focus on Mice and Rats

Ewa Domarecka [1] and Agnieszka J. Szczepek [1,2,*]

[1] Department of Otorhinolaryngology, Head and Neck Surgery, Charité-Universitätsmedizin Berlin, Corporate Member of Freie Universität Berlin and Humboldt Universität zu Berlin, 10117 Berlin, Germany
[2] Faculty of Medicine and Health Sciences, University of Zielona Gora, 65-046 Zielona Gora, Poland
* Correspondence: agnes.szczepek@charite.de

Abstract: Translational audiology research aims to transfer basic research findings into practical clinical applications. While animal studies provide essential knowledge for translational research, there is an urgent need to improve the reproducibility of data derived from these studies. Sources of variability in animal research can be grouped into three areas: animal, equipment, and experimental. To increase standardization in animal research, we developed universal recommendations for designing and conducting studies using a standard audiological method: auditory brainstem response (ABR). The recommendations are domain-specific and are intended to guide the reader through the issues that are important when applying for ABR approval, preparing for, and conducting ABR experiments. Better experimental standardization, which is the goal of these guidelines, is expected to improve the understanding and interpretation of results, reduce the number of animals used in preclinical studies, and improve the translation of knowledge to the clinic.

Keywords: auditory brainstem responses; ABR; translational audiology; experimental audiology; rodents

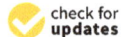

Citation: Domarecka, E.; Szczepek, A.J. Universal Recommendations on Planning and Performing the Auditory Brainstem Responses (ABR) with a Focus on Mice and Rats. *Audiol. Res.* **2023**, *13*, 441–458. https://doi.org/10.3390/audiolres13030039

Academic Editor: Andrea Ciorba

Received: 24 April 2023
Revised: 17 May 2023
Accepted: 29 May 2023
Published: 2 June 2023

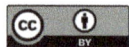

Copyright: © 2023 by the authors. Licensee MDPI, Basel, Switzerland. This article is an open access article distributed under the terms and conditions of the Creative Commons Attribution (CC BY) license (https://creativecommons.org/licenses/by/4.0/).

1. Introduction

Translational research aims to apply basic research findings to clinical practice. A translational project in audiology may involve pharmacological research, the development of non-pharmacological therapies, or disease monitoring [1]. The auditory brainstem response (ABR), also known as brainstem auditory evoked potentials (BAEPs) and short-latency auditory evoked potentials (SLAEPs), is a sensitive tool for determining the therapeutic potential of hearing loss therapies [2–5] and for diagnosing auditory nerve and brainstem dysfunction. Because of its objective nature, ABR is one of the few audiological tests that can be used for both human diagnostics and animal research. The results obtained from animal studies have translational potential and represent an essential step in developing therapeutics for otological disorders. According to the classification of translational research, such studies represent translational steps T0 (basic research aimed at understanding the pathological mechanisms of hearing loss or developing curative approaches) and reverse translation T1 (bedside to bench).

During an ABR, the electrical activity of auditory fibers evoked by an acoustic stimulus is recorded by electrodes placed on the skin (in humans) or subcutaneously (in animals) near the ear and auditory brainstem. ABRs consist of up to seven positive peaks, or waves, numbered from I to VII. In humans, wave I represents cochlear nerve activity (compound action potential, CAP), and wave II marks the exit of the cochlear nerve from the skull at the temporal bone. Waves III–V represent auditory brainstem activity [6]. Two key features of the ABR waves are their amplitudes and latencies. The amplitudes of the ABR waves provide information about the degree of synchronous action potential and the natural generators or modulators of the signal [6,7]. ABR latency reflects axonal conduction time and synaptic delay [6,8]. In clinical practice, ABR may help detect auditory neuropathies, retrocochlear lesions, or vestibular schwannomas [9]. It is also used for intraoperative monitoring to determine cochlear implant performance [10].

A great deal of insight into the development of ABR in animals has come from research on cats, and cats were the first group of animals in which ABR developmental changes were determined [11–13]. Depending on the research question, different animals, such as chickens, chinchillas, dogs, and bats, are used in experimental audiology. However, this paper will primarily focus on rats and mice, the two species most commonly used to study auditory responses using ABR (Figure 1).

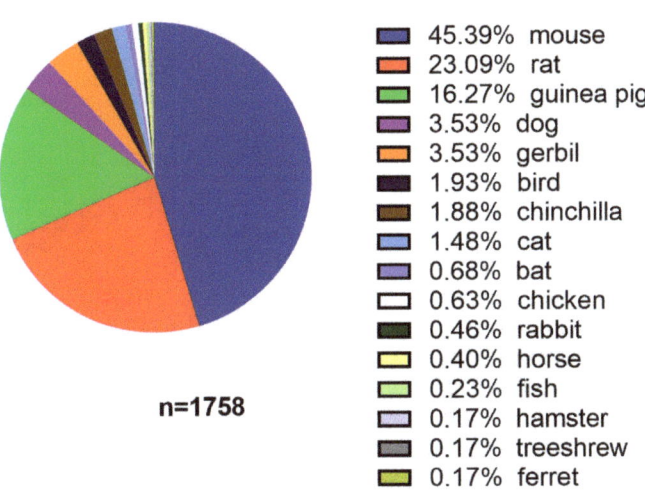

Figure 1. Usage of animal species in studies involving ABR published in PubMed between 2010 and 2022.

Rats are primarily used in pharmacological studies to develop new compounds [14]. Guinea pigs provide easy access to the cochlea and round window. Therefore, these animals are often used to research the round window approach of drug delivery and perilymph sampling [15]. Mice are used in genetic studies of inner ear pathology, although their hearing range differs from that of humans [16]. The gerbil's longevity (approximately three years) and resistance to developing middle ear disease make it an excellent model for age-related hearing loss [17].

Despite anatomical differences in the origins of ABR waves between species [18], the amplitude of wave I, which reflects the functional status of cochlear ribbon synapses and represents the functional integrity of auditory nerve fibers [19,20], is a sensitive marker of synaptopathy (recorded to suprathreshold transients) in both humans [21] and animals [22]. Wave V in humans probably corresponds to wave IV in animals [23].

Experimental ABR studies often yield significant results of potential clinical significance. However, data heterogeneity often precludes translation to the clinic. Data heterogeneity is related to several factors representing three domains: animal-, equipment-, and experiment-dependent. In the previous work, we analyzed the impact of each of these domains on the results of the ABR [24,25]. Here, we synthesized the knowledge on performing ABR in experimental animals to provide general recommendations. These recommendations consist of three parts: the planning of the experiment, the preparation of the ABR recordings, and the performance of the ABR recordings concerning three domains: animal-, equipment-, and experiment-related (Figure 2). Improving the reliability of results and minimizing experimental variability are the ultimate goals of the recommendations [26].

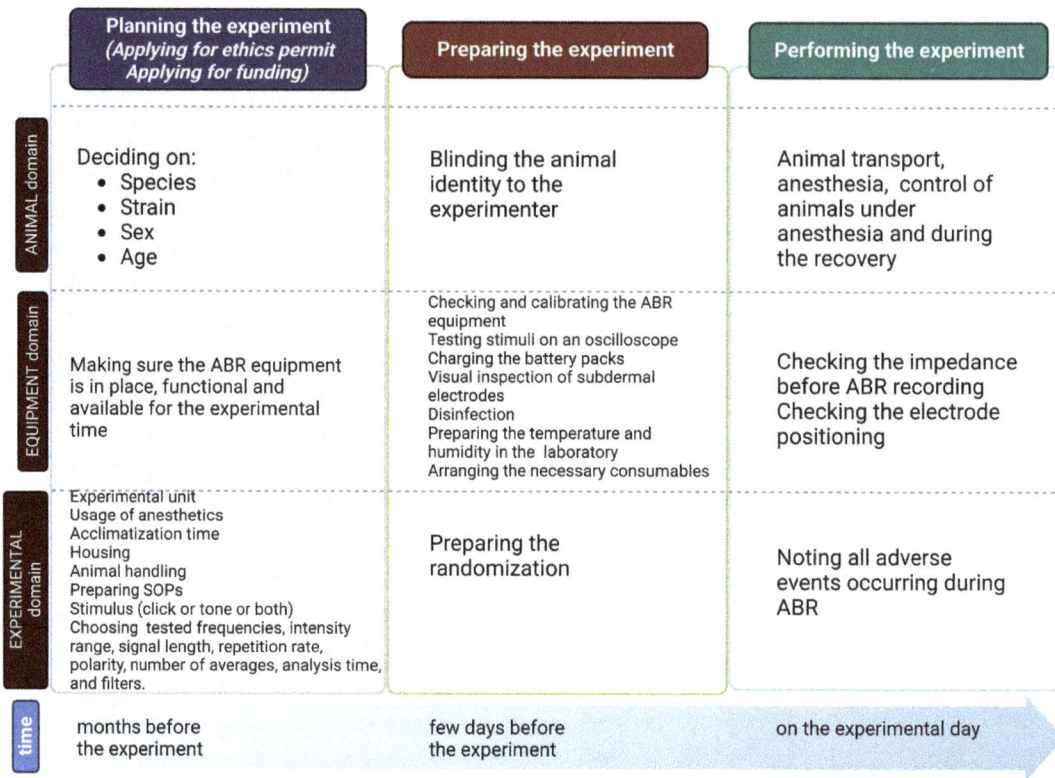

Figure 2. Schematic presentation of timelines and domains during the planning, preparation, and experimentation. Created with BioRender.com.

2. Planning the Experiment

The Experimental Design section refers to the outline of the experiment, which is usually part of the application to the ethics committee and/or the research grant application. After approval by the authorities, the only way to change this plan is to submit a supplemental application. Therefore, it is imperative at this stage to think through the project, discuss the procedure with laboratory members, and, if necessary, with the local veterinarian or animal facility representative. The more details addressed at this stage, the more time and peace of mind can be gained in conducting the experiments.

Because each country has different laws regarding the use of animals in research, no documents or links are given here. The investigator should find out how, when, and how to apply for an animal license in their institution. The first step in performing ABR on any animal is to obtain an animal use permit.

2.1. Planning the Experiment: Animals

This section addresses the species, strain (albino or pigmented), sex, age of the animals, and the number of animals included in the planned study. The animal's hearing range, size, and approximate life expectancy should be considered to select the appropriate species. The approximate hearing ranges of animals compared to humans are summarized in Figure 3. However, the choice of animal species may be influenced by factors other than hearing range, such as anatomical characteristics, life expectancy, or susceptibility to substances toxic to humans. For example, guinea pigs have larger tympanic bullae, which provide better access to the inner ear and are used in drug delivery studies by injection through the tympanic membrane or semicircular canal into the inner ear or for performing inner ear surgery. Due to their long lifespan (up to 20 years), chinchillas are not a standard model for age-related hearing loss [17], despite their hearing range being similar to humans. In the study of drug-induced hearing loss, a variety of species are used, and the different susceptibility of the species to ototoxins necessitates different dosage regimens [27]. Compared to guinea pigs, rats and mice are less susceptible to aminoglycoside-induced ototoxicity.

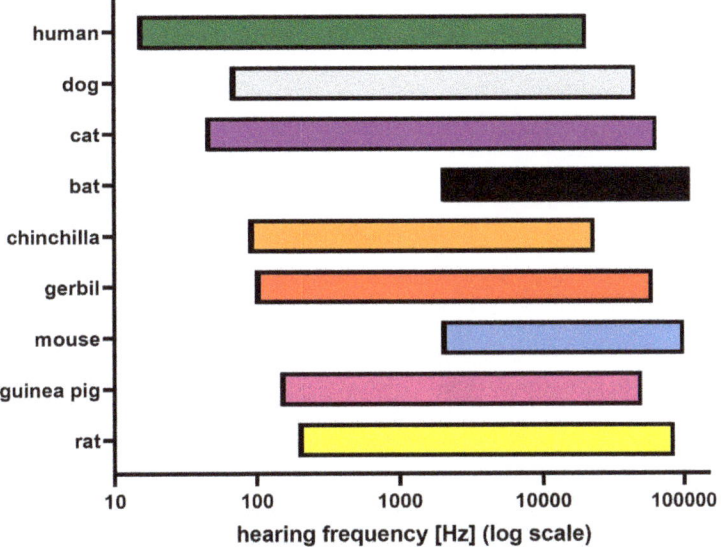

Figure 3. The hearing ranges of the most commonly used laboratory animals in ABR studies as compared to those of humans. Adapted from [28]. Due to the different paradigms that have been used to measure hearing range in different species, caution should be used in the interpretation of these results [29].

Both ABR thresholds and waveforms reflect strain differences [30,31]. For example, adult male (3–6 months old) Sprague-Dawley rats have a lower hearing threshold than Long-Evans rats (2–8 kHz). Adult (8-week) female Sprague-Dawley and Wistar rats had lower hearing thresholds below 26 kHz than Long-Evans and Lister Hooded rats [30]. Differences were observed between Sprague-Dawley and Wistar rats in the amplitude of wave IV: Sprague-Dawley rats had a higher amplitude than Wistars. Amplitude differences between Sprague-Dawley and Long-Evans strains were only observed when an 8 kHz tone burst elicited the ABR response. Sprague-Dawley rats have a higher amplitude of waves II, III, and IV than the Long-Evans strain [31]. Waves VI and VII are absent in animals [23].

Concerning laboratory mice, strain-dependent differences in the onset of age-related hearing loss (ARHL) have been reported (Table 1). Because CBA/CaJ mice have stable hearing (until 12–18 months of age), they are used in chronic ototoxic exposure experiments [32]. See elsewhere for more details on ARHL in mice [33].

Table 1. The onset of age-related hearing loss (ARHL or presbycusis) in selected mouse strains.

Mouse Strain	Onset of ARHL
C57Bl/6J	6 months [34]
CBA/J	20 months [32]
DBA/2J	3 weeks [35]
Balb/C	10 months [36]

Interestingly, unpigmented and pigmented animals have different inner ear morphologies [37–40]. Furthermore, melanin protected guinea pigs from noise-induced hearing loss [41]. Melanin precursors protected albino mice from age- and noise-induced hearing loss [42]. In addition, it was observed that the onset of age-related hearing loss differed between wild-type C57BL/6 and C57BL/6 Tyrc-2J albino mice, which was attributed to a melanin-dependent thinning of the striae, marginal cell loss, and a reduction of endocochlear potential [43].

There are behavioral differences between the strains of animals at the beginning and after the experimental treatment. Strain differences have been observed in male mice for sheltering behavior, locomotor activity, and behavior related to the dark/light phase [44]. Female mice from different strains have different sleeping habits [45]. Following noise exposure and salicylate administration, male Wistar rats developed more aggressive behavior than Sprague-Dawley rats [46]. Sometimes only female mice are used in a study because aggressive behavior may occur in large groups of unfamiliar male mice [47].

Sex bias has been identified as one of the factors contributing to poor translation in preclinical research [48]. Sex should be treated as a biological variable, and both sexes (equal numbers) should be included in the study design [48]. Exceptions to this are studies on the prevalence of the disease in only one sex, the performance of confirmatory experiments, or a pilot study. The justification should be provided in the study design if animals of only one sex are used. In audiology research, the effect of sex is reflected in differences in hearing ability [49], metabolism, and efficacy of medications [50]. Since the menstrual cycle affects the hearing thresholds of women, it should also be considered a confounding factor in animal studies [51]. Although sex affects the onset of presbyacusis, and male Fischer 344 rats exhibited age-related hearing loss earlier than female rats [52], differences in ABR latencies in the aging cochlea of CBA and C57 mice in males and females were not detected, which was attributed to minimal differences in brain size between the sexes [53]. Additionally, body mass and head/neck fat layer are confounding factors, as both are sex- and age-dependent [54,55]. Compared to females, male CBA/Ca mice are more susceptible to the adverse effects of a high-fat diet on body weight, metabolism, and hearing [56]. Because the subcutaneous fat layer has high electrical resistance and low conductance properties, and skin and muscle have low resistance and high conductance, this can result in high electrode impedance and affect ABR results [57].

The susceptibility of mice to noise and drug-induced hearing loss is age dependent. The noise susceptibility window in CBA/J mice begins at fifteen days of age and remains high until three months [58,59]. Consistent with these findings, young adult (1–2 months old) C57Blk/6J, CBA/CaJ, and Balb/CJ mice were more likely to develop noise-induced permanent threshold shifts than 5–7 month-old mice [60]. Similarly, susceptibility to ototoxic damage is age-dependent, and mice are most sensitive to drugs such as kanamycin during the first month of life [61,62]. Furthermore, susceptibility to drug-induced hearing loss depends on the exposure time and dose [63–65].

An essential step in preparing the experimental design is to decide how many animals will be included in each experimental group. A power analysis calculation should be performed to determine the sample size [66]. This mandatory calculation requires knowledge of effect size (significant difference between groups), standard deviation (only used for quantitative variables), power (probability of finding), the direction of effect, statistical test (simple vs. complex tests), and expected attrition of animal deaths [67]. An alternative method of sample size calculation is based on the law of diminishing returns—a technique used when it is difficult to specify an effect size [68]. The number of animals used in experiments should be kept as low as possible for ethical and practical reasons. Typically, 5–10 animals per group are used, which may not be sufficient for statistical analysis [69]. In such a case, a solution may be to perform pilot studies, sometimes with only one animal per group [66]. According to the ARRIVE guidelines, a justification for the number of animals included in the study should be reported.

Inclusion and exclusion criteria should be decided and not changed during the experiment. Examples of universal exclusion criteria include general animal health (abnormal appearance, tumors, otitis media, redness and swelling of local tissues, perforated tympanic membranes) and animal distress (appearance, behavior).

Finally, it is recommended that a Standard Operating Procedure (SOP) be prepared in the event of infectious contamination. Since the treatment given to one animal may affect other animals in the cage, it is good practice to consider all such animals as treated and include them in the same experimental unit.

2.2. Planning the Experiment: Equipment

An essential step is to ensure that the ABR equipment is in place, functional, and available for the duration of the experiment. There are several commercially available systems used in animal audiometry, manufactured by (in alphabetical order): ADInstruments (Castle Hill, Australia); Intelligent Hearing Systems (IHS, Miami, FL, USA); Interacoustic (Middelfart, Denmark); Neuro-Audio 0710 (Ivanovo, Russia); and Tucker Davis Technologies (TDT, Miami, FL, USA) [24]. Future studies should examine whether ABR results differ by device. Manufacturer's instructions for calibration and oscilloscope signal testing should be followed.

2.3. Planning the Experiment: Experiment

This domain includes stimulus design, the experimental unit, anesthetic use, acclimation time, housing, animal handling, and the possible influence of stress.

Although different commercial systems are used to perform small animal audiometry, the same stimulus parameters should be used for evoked ABR. The detailed protocol for performing ABR with TDT equipment and the IHS system [70] has been described elsewhere [71]. A video protocol showing ABR measurements in mice has also been described [72].

Depending on the purpose of the study, click or pure tone stimuli are used to elicit the ABR: tone burst stimuli are used to assess frequency-specific hearing, whereas click is used to assess high-frequency hearing, diagnose auditory nervous system disorders, or rapidly screen for hearing loss. The time required to complete the audiologic measurement is affected by either click or a tone burst.

The auditory stimulus consists of a sound spectrum, an intensity range, a signal length, a repetition rate, and a polarity. In addition, a number of averages, analysis time, and filters must be defined. Both the stimulus (e.g., type of stimulus, polarity) and the acquisition parameters (e.g., filters, analysis time) play a critical role in the quality of the ABR recording. Their effects are summarized in Table 2.

Either the entire hearing range or only a few selected frequencies are tested. The frequencies tested depend on the species. In mice and rats, typical test ranges include 4 kHz to 32 kHz, whereas, in guinea pigs, they range from 1 kHz to 18 kHz [73]. For gerbils, test ranges include 1 kHz to 8 kHz [74].

The click stimulus (a broadband signal) is characterized by a rapid onset and short duration. It activates more auditory nerve fibers and produces larger ABR amplitudes because its energy spans a broader frequency range than a tone burst [6]. The stimulus level can be independently adjusted. Three stimulus polarities are used: rarefaction, condensation, and alternating. Condensation clicks initially move the tympanic membrane inward, whereas rarefaction clicks move the tympanic membrane in the opposite direction [75]. The effect of the polarity of the ABR recordings has been discussed in the literature [23]. In humans with normal hearing, ABR recordings with either condensation or rarefaction polarity are nearly identical. Differences between click-evoked ABRs with condensing and rarefaction polarity were shown in cats [76]. For rarefaction clicks, the amplitude of wave I is greater. When recording is unreliable, alternating polarity (switching between condensation and rarefaction) can be used. Eliminating stimulus artifacts and cochlear microphonics makes Wave I more easily detectable [23].

The auditory stimulus can also be characterized by its repetition rate. As the stimulus repetition rate increases, amplitudes decrease, and latencies increase. Therefore, a slower stimulus rate will result in a more visible ABR waveform.

Windowing defines the shape of the tone burst signal, and it follows the rise, plateau, and fall of the stimulus. A stimulus that is too short will result in spectral splatter, while a stimulus that is too long will not produce a well-defined ABR (lower amplitude). Therefore, a 2-1-2 tone burst (two cycles of rise/fall time and one cycle of plateau time) is considered a compromise in humans [77]. In mice, 2.5 ms has been used in most studies [73].

In addition, noise reduction and averaging techniques are required for reliable amplitude assessment [78]. Noise can be environmental, instrumental, or generated within the body (physiological noise). Filters are used to improve the signal-to-noise ratio (SNR) [79]. A high-pass filter removes low-frequency noise, while a low-pass filter removes high-frequency noise [75]. Since electrophysiological signals are often plagued by noise from the power line (50 or 60 Hz and harmonics), a notch filter is used to eliminate this noise [80]. A detailed description of the use of filters has been provided by Cheveigné and Nelken [80]. Signal distribution/loudspeaker placement depends on the manufacturer's recommendations.

Because decreasing stimulus intensity results in longer latencies and lower amplitudes of ABR waves, 2–3 ABR traces should be collected at a near-threshold intensity to estimate the ABR threshold and correctly identify relevant peaks. In addition, low amplitude responses require more averages to verify ABR results. Since the ABR signal typically occurs in the 1 to 2.5 microvolt range, amplification is needed. A gain is used to remove the effect of hardware amplification of the response signal [73]. Use the value specified by the manufacturer.

Table 2. Factors influencing ABR recordings.

Factor	Definition	Influence on ABR Results	Suggestions Based on ABR User Guide
Ramp Number of Cycles (Rise-Plateau-Fall, e.g., 5 ms (2-1-2))	The number of sinusoidal waves in the rise, plateau, and fall portions of the tone burst's waveform. Only applicable for tone-burst	An increment in the rise time of the signal stimulus results in elongated absolute latencies [81]	mouse studies: mainly 2.5 ms
Repetition rate	Number of stimuli produced per second	Amplitude decrease with an increasing repetition rate of the stimuli—an increase in repetition rate results in an increase in ABR latencies.	21/s
Polarity	Crucial for initial stimulus presentation since it determines the way the sound pressure wave is presented [82]	Three stimulus polarities are used; i.e., rarefaction, condensation, and alternating. The latency of waves I, III, and V are shorter in response to the rarefaction click than the condensation click [83].	Rarefaction or alternating
Number of averages		Impact on the signal-to-noise ratio. The number of averages balances signal quality and minimalization of the time to complete testing.	The typical range of averages: 256–1024
Analysis time/ Recording window	A period following the stimulus is presented to the subject, during which the response is averaged and analyzed	Since decreasing stimulus intensity reduces the amplitude and increases latencies, the analysis time is extended to 15 ms to estimate the hearing threshold.	10 ms

Table 2. Cont.

Factor	Definition	Influence on ABR Results	Suggestions Based on ABR User Guide
Sampling rate	The average number of samples acquired per second		12 KHz
Artifact Rejection Threshold	The value defines the lowest level of electrophysiological activity, which contains excessive electric noise.	Clearer ABR response	
Filters	Use filters to separate signals based on their frequency, attenuating (reducing in amplitude) the unwanted frequency components and/or emphasizing the features that are important to us [79]	Filters make the presence or absence of the ABR responses more obvious since noise is filtered out.	Highpass filter: 300 Hz Lowpass filter: 3 kHz

Three main study designs are used in experimental audiology. The first type uses one ear as the experimental ear, while the contralateral ear is the control. This model is predominantly used in studies of ear surgery or the efficacy of drug administration. To use this model in studies of noise-induced hearing loss, an earplug must be used to protect one ear during noise exposure, while in studies of drug-induced hearing loss, the drug should be locally rather than systemically administered. In the second type of study, animals are divided into experimental and control groups. In the third type of study, all animals are examined at baseline and after treatment (before-after). This model ensures better identification of changes in ABR thresholds and waveforms by eliminating inter-animal differences and controlling for baseline variations.

When the purpose of the study is to estimate the effect of earlier treatment on hearing function, to determine whether hearing changes are gradually developing, and finally to test whether these changes are transient or permanent, the time course of recovery of ABR results is analyzed. One of the ways to assess this is to calculate the correlation factor (corF), which reflects the changes in waveform and amplitude before and after exposure to noise or toxic substances. High values (around 1) indicate the similarity of a waveform, whereas low values (around 0) reflect the loss of both waveform similarity and amplitude [84,85]. Depending on the experiment's length, the fat layer's thickness and the animals' age should be considered confounding factors.

Next, the number of animals to be tested daily with ABR should be determined. It is recommended to perform the audiological tests at the same time of the day to minimize the possible effects of diurnal rhythm since the function of the auditory system (both peripheral and central) is regulated by circadian mechanisms [86]. In addition, problems with anesthesia may prolong the measurement time.

The choice of an appropriate anesthetic is of great importance. Depending on laboratory capabilities and ethical requirements in a given country, inhalation gas or injectable drugs may be used. In the case of inhalation anesthesia, the anesthesia equipment should have been calibrated within the last 12 months. The local animal caretaker or veterinarian may be consulted for advice on the appropriate anesthetic and dosage. In most studies, isoflurane is used as an inhalation anesthetic, whereas ketamine/xylazine mixtures are used for injections. Technical details on the administration of isoflurane to animals can be found elsewhere [87]. Although the same drugs are used, different doses are applied, which affects the anesthetic conditions (working time and depth of anesthesia) [88] and explains the high heterogeneity of results. The advantages and disadvantages of using these anesthetics are summarized in Table 3.

Table 3. Advantages and disadvantages of using particular anesthetics for ABR studies.

Anesthetic	Sedation [73]	Drawbacks
Xylazine + Ketamine (i.p., i.m.)	Last ~45 min, the animal is awake after ~90 min from the initial injection. In male Wistar rats, complete sedation occurs in 10 min [89]	Requires proper restraining; rats anesthetized with this drug are more likely to develop corneal lesions than rats anesthetized with isoflurane, which is essential for long-term studies [90].
Isoflurane (inhalation)	Fast-acting, short-acting inhalation agent; the animal is usually fully sedated within 4–5 min. When the gas is removed, the animal wakes up very quickly.	Long-Evans rats anesthetized with isoflurane had higher hearing thresholds than rats anesthetized with ketamine/xylazine. Both click and tone thresholds were elevated, and the ABR response was worse [91,92].

Injectable anesthetics can be intraperitoneally, intramuscularly, or intravenously administered [93]. However, each type of injection requires proper restraint technique and has disadvantages, such as difficulty finding a superficial vein (intravenous), a high failure rate (intraperitoneal) [94,95], a less predictable route (subcutaneous) [96], or tissue reactions (intramuscular) [97]. Learning proper restraint techniques is recommended to avoid overdosing with injectable anesthetics. It is important to first assess the effects of anesthesia on an animal, to use healthy animals, to use drugs with a wide margin of safety, and to use comfortable syringes, such as those used to inject insulin in humans [98].

If ABR is to be recorded more than once, the SOP for recovery from anesthesia should be prepared.

At least one week of acclimatization should be allowed after transport to the animal facility to prevent the influence of stress on the experimental outcome. During this time, transport-induced metabolic and hormonal changes return to baseline [99]. The acclimation period should be extended if the day/night cycle is reversed.

The type and size of cages used should be appropriate to the number of animals housed per cage. Welfare assessments should be planned before, during, and after the experiment. The minimum cage size can be estimated based on the age of the animals when they are permanently removed from their home cage. Cage replacement should be avoided. If the animals are aggressive and must be separated from cage mates, the SOP should be prepared for such a situation.

An additional confounding factor in animal studies is stress, which has already been mentioned a number of times in this paper. Since both physical and psychological stress affect the hearing ability of animals [7], it is necessary to identify all possible stressors in the study design, such as environmental noise, handling, isolation, cage changes, and injections.

- Environmental noise can impact the hearing abilities of animals. Human activity is the primary source of environmental noise; therefore, all noise-generating activities inside the animal facility should be reduced to a minimum [100,101].
- The SOP describing the handling of animals should be prepared beforehand, and all unnecessary handling should be avoided. A handling tunnel or cupping without restraint in the open hand can minimize the anxiety of mice [102]. It is worth noting that the presence of men in breeding or experimental rooms is stressful for mice [103]. Animal behavior is also influenced by the animals' familiarity with the personnel involved in the experiment [104]. Importantly, the same breeds of animals purchased from different suppliers may respond to stress in various ways [105].
- Note: Experimenters should not wear scented cosmetics [106].

- Since cage changing is stressful for animals, cleaning cages should be planned in advance [106].
- In addition, social isolation can cause somatic reactions and should be avoided.
- Repeated intraperitoneal injections are also known to stress animals. Attention task performance was similar in rats chronically sham injected and chronically sham injected and restrained [107].

It is important to dedicate a person responsible for feeding and observing animals during the experiment. Abnormal posture, changes in motoric activity, reduced water and food intake (differences in the size of animals are a source of variability between animals), gait disturbance, erected hairs, weight loss, hypersalivation, abnormal licking, chewing movement, tremor, desensitization, moaning, and aggressive behavior should be observed and marked in the experimental protocol.

3. Preparing ABR Recordings

3.1. Preparing ABR Recordings: Animals

The experimenter should be blinded to the animal's identity (e.g., treated or untreated). Tips for improving study blinding have been described elsewhere [108]. Nevertheless, blinding (masking) is not always possible, e.g., when performing a comparative analysis of older and younger animals, as older animals are heavier and present alternation in body conditions compared to young animals. Based on ABR recording, noise-exposed animals are easily identified during the experiment [109].

3.2. Preparing ABR Recordings: Equipment

Two to three days before measurement, the system used to measure the ABR should be thoroughly checked and calibrated. Because calibration requires proper equipment, it should always be performed according to the manufacturer's instructions. In addition, an oscilloscope test should be performed to provide a visual representation of the shape or waveform of the signal. Again, follow the manufacturer's instructions.

Battery packs should be fully charged. Visual inspection of the subdermal electrodes should determine the need for replacement due to corrosion, blunting, bending, or other damage. The disinfectant should be prepared, and the experimental instruments should be disinfected or autoclaved. In addition, the environmental noise level should be determined by performing a saline test. See elsewhere for details [110].

The conditions (temperature, humidity) in the animal facility should be noted to mimic them as closely as possible in the experimental area (ABR room). The experimental area should be prepared to avoid unnecessary movements (gloves, syringes, etc., should be ready to be at hand).

3.3. Preparing ABR Recordings: Experiment

The random assignment of animals to experimental groups is necessary to minimize the effects of subjective bias. The PREPARE and ARRIVE guidelines identify randomization as mandatory in any animal study. Programs such as IBM SPSS Statistics, Prism GraphPad (www.graphpad.com/quickcalcs), randomizer.org, or the RandoMice tools can perform randomization [111]. Practical information on randomization can also be found on the ReproducibiliTeach YouTube channel (https://www.youtube.com/@reproducibiliteach, accessed on 19 April 2023).

4. Performing ABR

4.1. Performing ABR: Animals

This area covers animal transfer to the ABR research facility, anesthesia, and the monitoring of anesthetized animals.

After being transferred from the animal facility to the laboratory, animals should be allowed at least 15 min to acclimate. If possible, avoid changing cages during the transport and isolation of animals. Because small mammals (mice, rats, hamsters, guinea pigs, and rabbits) cannot regurgitate, it is not recommended that food be withheld before anesthesia—these animals should be provided with water and food ad libitum. However, in carnivores (e.g., dogs, cats, or ferrets) and insectivores (e.g., bats), food deprivation is mandatory as part of the preparation for anesthesia. Details can be found on the homepage of the Society for Laboratory Animal Science (https://www.gv-solas.de/?lang=en, accessed on 24 March 2023) or in a publication dedicated to that topic [112].

If injectable anesthesia is used, before removing the animal from the cage, it should be ensured that the animal is not exhibiting aggressive behavior. If so, wait until the animal has calmed down. Prepare an appropriate dose of anesthetic based on the animal's weight in a sterile vial or bottle (shake well before use). Mixed drugs should be protected from light and stored at room temperature on an experimental day. The rest of the drug or drugs mix or their waste should be disposed of according to local regulations—it equally regards the inhalation and non-inhalation drugs [113].

The most consistent and artifact-free ABR signals are obtained from stable anesthetized animals; otherwise, spontaneous muscle twitches over 100 times larger than the ABR may occur and completely overwhelm the signal. Applying ophthalmic ointment to both eyes is recommended to reduce the risk of corneal abrasions. Susceptibility to corneal injury is strain dependent [90].

An awake animal should not be housed with an anesthetized animal [114]. Five minutes after applying anesthesia (on average, usual time between the injection and loss of motor responses to noxious stimuli), check whether the animal is deeply anesthetized (eyelid reflex, toe reflex, tail flick reflex, nose, and vibrissae). For details on the depth and stages of anesthesia, please refer to a specific publication [115]. If the reflexes are still present, wait another 5 min, and if deep anesthesia cannot be confirmed after this time, review the protocol and refer to the SOP. Further action (additional injections, calling a veterinarian, returning the animal to the facility, or sacrificing the animal) depends on the country, ethical approval, and specific local regulations.

Once the animal is under deep anesthesia, the skin can be disinfected, and the electrodes subdermally placed. Care should be taken to ensure the electrodes are always placed in the same position. If the recording is repeated (recovery experiments), the position of the electrodes should be marked (e.g., by shaving the areas).

Transfer the animal to the ABR room. Perform an otoscopy to check the condition of the middle ear. Animals with ear canal or tympanic membrane abnormalities should be excluded from further experiments [24]. If necessary, remove the earwax.

During the anesthesia, the animal should be covered (e.g., with paper towels—do not use electric heating pads as most of them may interfere with the ABR recording) to keep it warm. Monitor and maintain the animal's body temperature to prevent the disruption of thermoregulation and eliminate the body temperature's effect on ABR records. A temperature decrease of 0.5 °C or more may significantly alter ABR latencies and amplitudes [116,117]. Monitor the anesthesia. The duration of anesthesia depends on the species and the anesthetic used. For example, the duration of anesthesia induced by ketamine + xylazine is typically 30 to 45 min. After this time, half the dose may be administered as needed.

Do not leave an anesthetized animal unattended during the recovery process. Keep the animal warm by covering it. Return the animal to its cage as soon as it begins to move and allow it to recover fully. Record the recovery time in the log. Recording food and water consumption in the pre- and postoperative periods is good practice to confirm that animals are in a regular physical state after recovery from anesthesia. Intake of both will be reduced if the animal is in pain [98].

4.2. Performing ABR: Equipment

Since significant amplitude variations can be related to electrode impedance, the impedance should be checked before ABR recording. Impedance >3 kΩ results in lower artifact suppression, lower recording quality, and incorrect threshold recognition at the sound pressure level of roughly 20 dB. Furthermore, the resistance between the recording and active electrodes should be tested. Since the placement of the reference electrode affects ABR recordings, carefully check the position of the needle electrodes [118]. A reference electrode is placed behind the ipsilateral ear. An active electrode is commonly placed on the vertex (base of the skull), and a ground electrode is placed at the back, hind hip, or base of the tail. Since the ABR is recorded from electrodes placed on the vertex and the electrode behind the ipsilateral ear [75], do not forget to change the reference electrode when switching between ears (the electrode's position depends on the ear, which is measured; Figure 4).

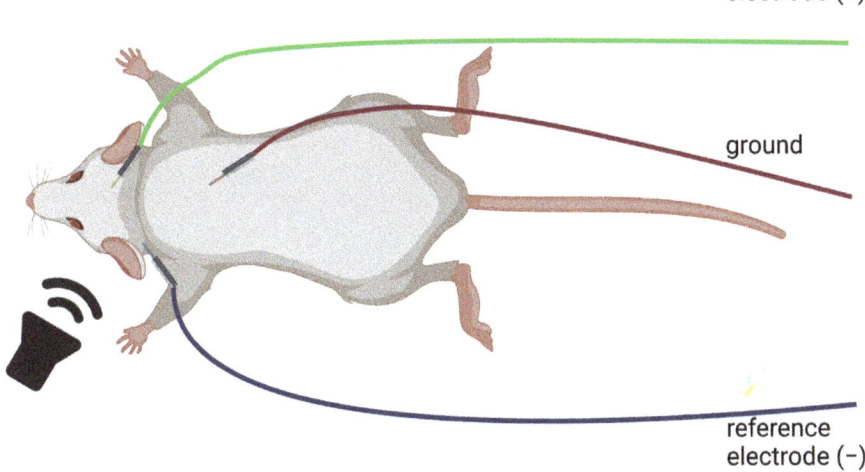

Figure 4. Example of electrode positioning for ABR. Created with BioRender.com.

The impact of the animal fat layer in the head/neck region on impedance has been previously discussed [24]. Since the ABR signal typically occurs in the 1–2.5 microVolt range, removing cables, wires, and noise generators from the test area is crucial.

Start the measurement. Correctly identifying the waveform, especially in the abnormal waveform, is challenging. Because waves II, IV, VI, and VII are inconsistent in humans, they are generally not considered for clinical interpretation [23]. To improve wave identification, an automated tool for ABR waves has been developed [119], which was possible because ABR has a predictable pattern. Therefore, time intervals for each wave were used to find the local extrema of the waveforms. The same rules are used to identify waves in animals. First, wave I is identified, and then the rest of the waves are identified. Depending on the literature, either wave II or III is the most prominent in rodents. The automatically detected ABR threshold is similar to the visually detected threshold [120].

At the end of the recording, remove the electrodes, disinfect them, and store them in a sterile container (record the number of times the electrodes were used in the protocol). Ensure that all recorded traces are saved for further analysis (.txt files can be uploaded into an Excel file) [70].

4.3. Performing ABR: Experiment

Any adverse events during the ABR recording should be noted in the protocol. The reasons for excluding an animal from the analysis should be recorded in the protocol. Room temperature variations should also be considered a confounding factor [121]. Detailed experimental records can help quickly identify the source of variability between animals, especially differences between animals during the same experiments [65]. A sex-specific analysis should be performed if male and female animals were included in the study. Data analysis should be based on the experimental design.

4.4. Protocols

The published research performed with ABR usually contains respective protocols. However, manuscripts focused on detailed ABR protocols have also been published in peer-reviewed journals, and we list them in Table 4 below.

Table 4. Publications focused on ABR protocols.

Title	Publication Year	Species	Ref.
Measurement of the auditory brainstem response (ABR) to study auditory sensitivity in mice	2006	mice	[122]
Using the Auditory Brainstem Response (ABR) to Determine Sensitivity of Hearing in Mutant Mice	2011	mice	[123]
Mouse Auditory Brainstem Response Testing	2016	mice	[114]
Data Acquisition and Analysis In Brainstem Evoked Response Audiometry In Mice	2019	mice	[72]
Protocol for assessing auditory brainstem response in mice using a four-channel recording system	2022	mice	[124]
Auditory brainstem response (ABR) measurements in small mammals," in Developmental, Physiological, and Functional Neurobiology of the Inner Ear	2022	mice (suggested application also for rats, hamsters, and bats)	[71]

5. Conclusions

ABR is a non-invasive technique that measures electrical potential reflecting neural activity in the auditory pathway and can be used to identify markers of different auditory conditions. Improving data reproducibility during preclinical studies is necessary to translate animal research into the clinic. Such improvement can be achieved by standardizing the design, conducting experiments, and reporting all information in publications according to the ARRIVE guidelines [125]. In addition, the management of sources of variability should be addressed in every publication [126], leading to a better understanding and improved translation of the results obtained and reducing the number of experimental animals used.

Author Contributions: Conceptualization, A.J.S. and E.D.; methodology, E.D.; software, investigation, E.D. and A.J.S.; resources, A.J.S.; writing—original draft preparation, E.D.; writing—review and editing, E.D. and A.J.S.; visualization, A.J.S.; supervision, A.J.S.; project administration, A.J.S. All authors have read and agreed to the published version of the manuscript.

Funding: This research received no external funding.

Data Availability Statement: No new data were created or analyzed in this study. Data sharing is not applicable to this article.

Conflicts of Interest: The authors declare no conflict of interest.

References

1. Szczepek, A.J.; Domarecka, E.; Olze, H. Translational Research in Audiology: Presence in the Literature. *Audiol. Res.* **2022**, *12*, 674–679. [CrossRef] [PubMed]
2. Vlajkovic, S.M.; Chang, H.; Paek, S.Y.; Chi, H.H.; Sreebhavan, S.; Telang, R.S.; Tingle, M.; Housley, G.D.; Thorne, P.R. Adenosine amine congener as a cochlear rescue agent. *BioMed Res. Int.* **2014**, *2014*, 841489. [CrossRef] [PubMed]
3. Choi, C.H.; Chen, K.; Du, X.; Floyd, R.A.; Kopke, R.D. Effects of delayed and extended antioxidant treatment on acute acoustic trauma. *Free Radic. Res.* **2011**, *45*, 1162–1172. [CrossRef] [PubMed]
4. Ewert, D.; Hu, N.; Du, X.; Li, W.; West, M.B.; Choi, C.H.; Floyd, R.; Kopke, R.D. HPN-07, a free radical spin trapping agent, protects against functional, cellular and electrophysiological changes in the cochlea induced by acute acoustic trauma. *PLoS ONE* **2017**, *12*, e0183089. [CrossRef]
5. Wang, J.; Tian, K.Y.; Fang, Y.; Chang, H.M.; Han, Y.N.; Chen, F.Q. Sulforaphane attenuates cisplatin-induced hearing loss by inhibiting histone deacetylase expression. *Int. J. Immunopathol. Pharmacol.* **2021**, *35*, 20587384211034086. [CrossRef] [PubMed]

6. Eggermont, J.J. Chapter 30-Auditory brainstem response. In *Handbook of Clinical Neurology*; Levin, K.H., Chauvel, P., Eds.; Elsevier: Amsterdam, The Netherlands, 2019; Volume 160, pp. 451–464.
7. Szczepek, A.J.; Dietz, G.P.H.; Reich, U.; Hegend, O.; Olze, H.; Mazurek, B. Differences in Stress-Induced Modulation of the Auditory System Between Wistar and Lewis Rats. *Front. Neurosci.* **2018**, *12*, 828. [CrossRef]
8. Fabiani, M.; Sohmer, H.; Tait, C.; Gafni, M.; Kinarti, R. A functional measure of brain activity: Brain stem transmission time. *Electroencephalogr. Clin. Neurophysiol.* **1979**, *47*, 483–491. [CrossRef]
9. Rupa, V.; Job, A.; George, M.; Rajshekhar, V. Cost-effective initial screening for vestibular schwannoma: Auditory brainstem response or magnetic resonance imaging? *Otolaryngol. Head. Neck Surg.* **2003**, *128*, 823–828. [CrossRef]
10. Ren, W.; Ji, F.; Zeng, J.; Zhao, H. Intra-operative hearing monitoring methods in middle ear surgeries. *J. Otol.* **2016**, *11*, 178–184. [CrossRef]
11. Walsh, E.J.; McGee, J.; Javel, E. Development of auditory-evoked potentials in the cat. I. Onset of response and development of sensitivity. *J. Acoust. Soc. Am.* **1986**, *79*, 712–724. [CrossRef]
12. Walsh, E.J.; McGee, J.; Javel, E. Development of auditory-evoked potentials in the cat. III. Wave amplitudes. *J. Acoust. Soc. Am.* **1986**, *79*, 745–754. [CrossRef] [PubMed]
13. Walsh, E.J.; McGee, J.; Javel, E. Development of auditory-evoked potentials in the cat. II. Wave latencies. *J. Acoust. Soc. Am.* **1986**, *79*, 725–744. [CrossRef]
14. Cederroth, C.R.; Dyhrfjeld-Johnsen, J.; Langguth, B. An update: Emerging drugs for tinnitus. *Expert Opin. Emerg. Drugs* **2018**, *23*, 251–260. [CrossRef] [PubMed]
15. Naert, G.; Pasdelou, M.P.; Le Prell, C.G. Use of the guinea pig in studies on the development and prevention of acquired sensorineural hearing loss, with an emphasis on noise. *J. Acoust. Soc. Am.* **2019**, *146*, 3743. [CrossRef] [PubMed]
16. Ohlemiller, K.K.; Jones, S.M.; Johnson, K.R. Application of Mouse Models to Research in Hearing and Balance. *J. Assoc. Res. Otolaryngol.* **2016**, *17*, 493–523. [CrossRef]
17. Boettcher, F.A. Presbyacusis and the auditory brainstem response. *J. Speech Lang. Hear. Res.* **2002**, *45*, 1249–1261. [CrossRef]
18. Laumen, G.; Ferber, A.T.; Klump, G.M.; Tollin, D.J. The Physiological Basis and Clinical Use of the Binaural Interaction Component of the Auditory Brainstem Response. *Ear Hear.* **2016**, *37*, e276–e290. [CrossRef]
19. Sergeyenko, Y.; Lall, K.; Liberman, M.C.; Kujawa, S.G. Age-related cochlear synaptopathy: An early-onset contributor to auditory functional decline. *J. Neurosci. Off. J. Soc. Neurosci.* **2013**, *33*, 13686–13694. [CrossRef]
20. Kujawa, S.G.; Liberman, M.C. Adding insult to injury: Cochlear nerve degeneration after "temporary" noise-induced hearing loss. *J. Neurosci. Off. J. Soc. Neurosci.* **2009**, *29*, 14077–14085. [CrossRef]
21. Bramhall, N.F.; Konrad-Martin, D.; McMillan, G.P.; Griest, S.E. Auditory Brainstem Response Altered in Humans with Noise Exposure Despite Normal Outer Hair Cell Function. *Ear Hear.* **2017**, *38*, e1–e12. [CrossRef]
22. Kujawa, S.G.; Liberman, M.C. Synaptopathy in the noise-exposed and aging cochlea: Primary neural degeneration in acquired sensorineural hearing loss. *Hear. Res.* **2015**, *330*, 191–199. [CrossRef] [PubMed]
23. Markand, O.N. Brainstem Auditory Evoked Potentials. In *Clinical Evoked Potentials: An. Illustrated Manual*; Markand, O.N., Ed.; Springer International Publishing: Cham, Switzerland, 2020; pp. 25–82.
24. Domarecka, E.; Kalcioglu, M.T.; Mutlu, A.; Özgür, A.; Smit, J.; Olze, H.; Szczepek, A.J. Reporting Data on Auditory Brainstem Responses (ABR) in Rats: Recommendations Based on Review of Experimental Protocols and Literature. *Brain Sci.* **2021**, *11*, 1596. [CrossRef] [PubMed]
25. Domarecka, E.; Olze, H.; Szczepek, A.J. Auditory Brainstem Responses (ABR) of Rats during Experimentally Induced Tinnitus: Literature Review. *Brain Sci.* **2020**, *10*, 901. [CrossRef]
26. Bracken, M.B. Why animal studies are often poor predictors of human reactions to exposure. *J. R. Soc. Med.* **2009**, *102*, 120–122. [CrossRef] [PubMed]
27. Lin, X.; Luo, J.; Tan, J.; Yang, L.; Wang, M.; Li, P. Experimental animal models of drug-induced sensorineural hearing loss: A narrative review. *Ann. Transl. Med.* **2021**, *9*, 1393. [CrossRef] [PubMed]
28. Heffner, H.E.; Heffner, R.S. Hearing ranges of laboratory animals. *J. Am. Assoc. Lab. Anim. Sci.* **2007**, *46*, 20–22.
29. Popper, A.N.; Fay, R.R. *Comparative Studies of Hearing in Vertebrates*; Springer Science & Business Media: New York, NY, USA, 2012.
30. Koch, L.; Gaese, B.H.; Nowotny, M. Strain Comparison in Rats Differentiates Strain-Specific from More General Correlates of Noise-Induced Hearing Loss and Tinnitus. *J. Assoc. Res. Otolaryngol.* **2022**, *23*, 59–73. [CrossRef]
31. Overbeck, G.W.; Church, M.W. Effects of tone burst frequency and intensity on the auditory brainstem response (ABR) from albino and pigmented rats. *Hear. Res.* **1992**, *59*, 129–137. [CrossRef]
32. Sha, S.H.; Kanicki, A.; Dootz, G.; Talaska, A.E.; Halsey, K.; Dolan, D.; Altschuler, R.; Schacht, J. Age-related auditory pathology in the CBA/J mouse. *Hear. Res.* **2008**, *243*, 87–94. [CrossRef]
33. Zheng, Q.Y.; Johnson, K.R.; Erway, L.C. Assessment of hearing in 80 inbred strains of mice by ABR threshold analyses. *Hear. Res.* **1999**, *130*, 94–107. [CrossRef]
34. Li, H.S.; Borg, E. Age-related loss of auditory sensitivity in two mouse genotypes. *Acta Otolaryngol.* **1991**, *111*, 827–834. [CrossRef] [PubMed]
35. Yang, L.; Zhang, H.; Han, X.; Zhao, X.; Hu, F.; Li, P.; Xie, G.; Gao, L.; Cheng, L.; Song, X.; et al. Attenuation of hearing loss in DBA/2J mice by anti-apoptotic treatment. *Hear. Res.* **2015**, *327*, 109–116. [CrossRef] [PubMed]

36. Willott, J.F.; Turner, J.G.; Carlson, S.; Ding, D.; Seegers Bross, L.; Falls, W.A. The BALB/c mouse as an animal model for progressive sensorineural hearing loss. *Hear. Res.* **1998**, *115*, 162–174. [CrossRef] [PubMed]
37. Jin, Z.; Mannström, P.; Skjönsberg, A.; Järlebark, L.; Ulfendahl, M. Auditory function and cochlear morphology in the German waltzing guinea pig. *Hear. Res.* **2006**, *219*, 74–84. [CrossRef] [PubMed]
38. Hoshino, T.; Mizuta, K.; Gao, J.; Araki, S.; Araki, K.; Takeshita, T.; Wu, R.; Morita, H. Cochlear findings in the white spotting (Ws) rat. *Hear. Res.* **2000**, *140*, 145–156. [CrossRef]
39. Heid, S.; Hartmann, R.; Klinke, R. A model for prelingual deafness, the congenitally deaf white cat—Population statistics and degenerative changes. *Hear. Res.* **1998**, *115*, 101–112. [CrossRef]
40. Mair, I.W. Hereditary deafness in the dalmatian dog. *Arch. Oto-Rhino-Laryngol.* **1976**, *212*, 1–14. [CrossRef]
41. Xiong, M.; He, Q.; Lai, H.; Wang, J. Oxidative stress in spiral ganglion cells of pigmented and albino guinea pigs exposed to impulse noise. *Acta Otolaryngol.* **2011**, *131*, 914–920. [CrossRef]
42. Murillo-Cuesta, S.; Contreras, J.; Zurita, E.; Cediel, R.; Cantero, M.; Varela-Nieto, I.; Montoliu, L. Melanin precursors prevent premature age-related and noise-induced hearing loss in albino mice. *Pigment. Cell Melanoma Res.* **2010**, *23*, 72–83. [CrossRef]
43. Ohlemiller, K.K.; Rice, M.E.; Lett, J.M.; Gagnon, P.M. Absence of strial melanin coincides with age-associated marginal cell loss and endocochlear potential decline. *Hear. Res.* **2009**, *249*, 1–14. [CrossRef]
44. Loos, M.; Koopmans, B.; Aarts, E.; Maroteaux, G.; van der Sluis, S.; Verhage, M.; Smit, A.B. Sheltering behavior and locomotor activity in 11 genetically diverse common inbred mouse strains using home-cage monitoring. *PLoS ONE* **2014**, *9*, e108563. [CrossRef] [PubMed]
45. Koehl, M.; Battle, S.E.; Turek, F.W. Sleep in female mice: A strain comparison across the estrous cycle. *Sleep* **2003**, *26*, 267–272. [CrossRef] [PubMed]
46. Zheng, Y.; Hamilton, E.; McNamara, E.; Smith, P.F.; Darlington, C.L. The effects of chronic tinnitus caused by acoustic trauma on social behaviour and anxiety in rats. *Neuroscience* **2011**, *193*, 143–153. [CrossRef]
47. Heinla, I.; Åhlgren, J.; Vasar, E.; Voikar, V. Behavioural characterization of C57BL/6N and BALB/c female mice in social home cage—Effect of mixed housing in complex environment. *Physiol. Behav.* **2018**, *188*, 32–41. [CrossRef]
48. Karp, N.A.; Reavey, N. Sex bias in preclinical research and an exploration of how to change the status quo. *Br. J. Pharmacol.* **2019**, *176*, 4107–4118. [CrossRef]
49. Souza, D.D.S.; Luckwu, B.; Andrade, W.T.L.; Pessoa, L.S.F.; Nascimento, J.A.D.; Rosa, M. Variation in the Hearing Threshold in Women during the Menstrual Cycle. *Int. Arch. Otorhinolaryngol.* **2017**, *21*, 323–328. [CrossRef] [PubMed]
50. Anderson, G.D. Sex and racial differences in pharmacological response: Where is the evidence? Pharmacogenetics, pharmacokinetics, and pharmacodynamics. *J. Womens Health* **2005**, *14*, 19–29. [CrossRef] [PubMed]
51. Marcondes, F.K.; Bianchi, F.J.; Tanno, A.P. Determination of the estrous cycle phases of rats: Some helpful considerations. *Braz. J. Biol.* **2002**, *62*, 609–614. [CrossRef]
52. Balogová, Z.; Popelář, J.; Chiumenti, F.; Chumak, T.; Burianová, J.S.; Rybalko, N.; Syka, J. Age-Related Differences in Hearing Function and Cochlear Morphology between Male and Female Fischer 344 Rats. *Front. Aging Neurosci.* **2017**, *9*, 428. [CrossRef]
53. Hunter, K.P.; Willott, J.F. Aging and the auditory brainstem response in mice with severe or minimal presbycusis. *Hear. Res.* **1987**, *30*, 207–218. [CrossRef]
54. Virgen-Ortiz, A.; Apolinar-Iribe, A.; Muñiz, J. Gender-effect on the contractile properties of skeletal muscle in streptozotocin-induced diabetic rats. *J. Musculoskelet. Neuronal Interact.* **2018**, *18*, 255–261. [PubMed]
55. Quirós Cognuck, S.; Reis, W.L.; Silva, M.; Debarba, L.K.; Mecawi, A.S.; de Paula, F.J.A.; Rodrigues Franci, C.; Elias, L.L.K.; Antunes-Rodrigues, J. Sex differences in body composition, metabolism-related hormones, and energy homeostasis during aging in Wistar rats. *Physiol. Rep.* **2020**, *8*, e14597. [CrossRef] [PubMed]
56. Kim, S.J.; Gajbhiye, A.; Lyu, A.R.; Kim, T.H.; Shin, S.A.; Kwon, H.C.; Park, Y.H.; Park, M.J. Sex differences in hearing impairment due to diet-induced obesity in CBA/Ca mice. *Biol. Sex. Differ.* **2023**, *14*, 10. [CrossRef] [PubMed]
57. Petrofsky, J.; Schwab, E. A re-evaluation of modelling of the current flow between electrodes: Consideration of blood flow and wounds. *J. Med. Eng. Technol.* **2007**, *31*, 62–74. [CrossRef] [PubMed]
58. Henry, K.R. Influence of genotype and age on noise-induced auditory losses. *Behav. Genet.* **1982**, *12*, 563–573. [CrossRef]
59. Henry, K.R. Lifelong susceptibility to acoustic trauma: Changing patterns of cochlear damage over the life span of the mouse. *Audiology* **1983**, *22*, 372–383. [CrossRef]
60. Ohlemiller, K.K.; Wright, J.S.; Heidbreder, A.F. Vulnerability to noise-induced hearing loss in 'middle-aged' and young adult mice: A dose-response approach in CBA, C57BL, and BALB inbred strains. *Hear. Res.* **2000**, *149*, 239–247. [CrossRef]
61. Henry, K.R.; Chole, R.A.; McGinn, M.D.; Frush, D.P. Increased ototoxicity in both young and old mice. *Arch. Otolaryngol.* **1981**, *107*, 92–95. [CrossRef]
62. Prieve, B.A.; Yanz, J.L. Age-dependent changes in susceptibility to ototoxic hearing loss. *Acta Otolaryngol.* **1984**, *98*, 428–438. [CrossRef]
63. Bielefeld, E.C.; Gonzalez, A.; DeBacker, J.R. Changing the time intervals between cisplatin cycles alter its ototoxic side effect. *Hear. Res.* **2021**, *404*, 108204. [CrossRef]
64. Soulban, G.; Smolensky, M.H.; Yonovitz, A. Gentamicin-induced chronotoxicity: Use of body temperature as a circadian marker rhythm. *Chronobiol. Int.* **1990**, *7*, 393–402. [CrossRef] [PubMed]

65. Yonovitz, A.; Fisch, J.E. Circadian rhythm dependent kanamycin-induced hearing loss in rodents assessed by auditory brainstem responses. *Acta Otolaryngol.* **1991**, *111*, 1006–1012. [CrossRef] [PubMed]
66. Festing, M.F.; Altman, D.G. Guidelines for the design and statistical analysis of experiments using laboratory animals. *Ilar. J.* **2002**, *43*, 244–258. [CrossRef] [PubMed]
67. Charan, J.; Kantharia, N.D. How to calculate sample size in animal studies? *J. Pharmacol. Pharmacother.* **2013**, *4*, 303–306. [CrossRef]
68. Mead, R. *The Design of Experiments: Statistical Principles for Practical Applications*; Cambridge University Press: New York, NY, USA, 1988; 620p.
69. Ricci, C.; Baumgartner, J.; Malan, L.; Smuts, C.M. Determining sample size adequacy for animal model studies in nutrition research: Limits and ethical challenges of ordinary power calculation procedures. *Int. J. Food Sci. Nutr.* **2020**, *71*, 256–264. [CrossRef]
70. Ordiway, G.; McDonnell, M.; Mohan, S.; Sanchez, J.T. Evaluation of Auditory Brainstem Response in Chicken Hatchlings. *J. Vis. Exp.* **2022**, *182*, e63477. [CrossRef]
71. Kim, Y.H.; Schrode, K.M.; Lauer, A.M. Auditory brainstem response (ABR) measurements in small mammals. In *Developmental, Physiological, and Functional Neurobiology of the Inner Ear*; Humana: New York, NY, USA, 2022; pp. 357–375.
72. Lundt, A.; Soos, J.; Henseler, C.; Arshaad, M.I.; Müller, R.; Ehninger, D.; Hescheler, J.; Sachinidis, A.; Broich, K.; Wormuth, C.; et al. Data Acquisition and Analysis in Brainstem Evoked Response Audiometry in Mice. *J. Vis. Exp.* **2019**, *147*, e59200. [CrossRef]
73. Tucker-Davis-Technologies. ABR User Guide. Available online: https://www.tdt.com/files/manuals/ABRGuide.pdf (accessed on 9 February 2023).
74. Lanaia, V.; Tziridis, K.; Schulze, H. Salicylate-Induced Changes in Hearing Thresholds in Mongolian Gerbils Are Correlated with Tinnitus Frequency but Not with Tinnitus Strength. *Front. Behav. Neurosci.* **2021**, *15*, 698516. [CrossRef]
75. Moller, A.R. *Hearing: Anatomy, Physiology, and Disorders of the Auditory System*; Elsevier Science: Amsterdam, The Netherlands, 2006.
76. Melcher, J.R.; Knudson, I.M.; Fullerton, B.C.; Guinan, J.J., Jr.; Norris, B.E.; Kiang, N.Y. Generators of the brainstem auditory evoked potential in cat. I. An experimental approach to their identification. *Hear. Res.* **1996**, *93*, 1–27. [CrossRef]
77. Canale, A.; Dagna, F.; Lacilla, M.; Piumetto, E.; Albera, R. Relationship between pure tone audiometry and tone burst auditory brainstem response at low frequencies gated with Blackman window. *Eur. Arch. Oto-Rhino-Laryngol.* **2012**, *269*, 781–785. [CrossRef]
78. Burkard, R.; Secor, C. Overview of auditory evoked potentials. In *Handbook of Clinical Audiology*; Julet, T.L., Ed.; Lippincott Williams and Wilkins: Baltimore, MD, USA, 2002; pp. 233–248.
79. Burgess, R.C. Filtering of neurophysiologic signals. *Handb. Clin. Neurol.* **2019**, *160*, 51–65. [CrossRef]
80. De Cheveigné, A.; Nelken, I. Filters: When, Why, and How (Not) to Use Them. *Neuron* **2019**, *102*, 280–293. [CrossRef] [PubMed]
81. Fausti, S.A.; Gray, P.S.; Frey, R.H.; Mitchell, C.R. Rise time and center-frequency effects on auditory brainstem responses to high-frequency tone bursts. *J. Am. Acad. Audiol.* **1991**, *2*, 24–31. [PubMed]
82. Hall, J.W. *Handbook of Auditory Evoked Responses*; Allyn & Bacon: Boston, MA, USA, 1992.
83. Fowler, C.G. Effects of stimulus phase on the normal auditory brainstem response. *J. Speech Hear. Res.* **1992**, *35*, 167–174. [CrossRef] [PubMed]
84. Singer, W.; Zuccotti, A.; Jaumann, M.; Lee, S.C.; Panford-Walsh, R.; Xiong, H.; Zimmermann, U.; Franz, C.; Geisler, H.S.; Köpschall, I.; et al. Noise-induced inner hair cell ribbon loss disturbs central arc mobilization: A novel molecular paradigm for understanding tinnitus. *Mol. Neurobiol.* **2013**, *47*, 261–279. [CrossRef]
85. Bing, D.; Lee, S.C.; Campanelli, D.; Xiong, H.; Matsumoto, M.; Panford-Walsh, R.; Wolpert, S.; Praetorius, M.; Zimmermann, U.; Chu, H.; et al. Cochlear NMDA receptors as a therapeutic target of noise-induced tinnitus. *Cell. Physiol. Biochem.* **2015**, *35*, 1905–1923. [CrossRef]
86. Cederroth, C.; Gachon, F.; Canlon, B. Time to listen: Circadian impact on auditory research. *Curr. Opin. Physiol.* **2020**, *18*, 95–99. [CrossRef]
87. Greenfield, E.A. Administering Anesthesia to Mice, Rats, and Hamsters. *Cold Spring Harb. Protoc.* **2019**, *2019*, 457–459. [CrossRef]
88. Xu, Q.; Ming, Z.; Dart, A.M.; Du, X.J. Optimizing dosage of ketamine and xylazine in murine echocardiography. *Clin. Exp. Pharmacol. Physiol.* **2007**, *34*, 499–507. [CrossRef]
89. Albrecht, M.; Henke, J.; Tacke, S.; Markert, M.; Guth, B. Effects of isoflurane, ketamine-xylazine and a combination of medetomidine, midazolam and fentanyl on physiological variables continuously measured by telemetry in Wistar rats. *BMC Vet. Res.* **2014**, *10*, 198. [CrossRef]
90. Turner, P.V.; Albassam, M.A. Susceptibility of rats to corneal lesions after injectable anesthesia. *Comp. Med.* **2005**, *55*, 175–182. [PubMed]
91. Turner, J.G.; Larsen, D. Effects of noise exposure on development of tinnitus and hyperacusis: Prevalence rates 12 months after exposure in middle-aged rats. *Hear. Res.* **2016**, *334*, 30–36. [CrossRef] [PubMed]
92. Ouyang, J.; Pace, E.; Lepczyk, L.; Kaufman, M.; Zhang, J.; Perrine, S.A.; Zhang, J. Blast-Induced Tinnitus and Elevated Central Auditory and Limbic Activity in Rats: A Manganese-Enhanced MRI and Behavioral Study. *Sci. Rep.* **2017**, *7*, 4852. [CrossRef] [PubMed]
93. Ritschl, L.M.; Fichter, A.M.; Häberle, S.; von Bomhard, A.; Mitchell, D.A.; Wolff, K.D.; Mücke, T. Ketamine-Xylazine Anesthesia in Rats: Intraperitoneal versus Intravenous Administration Using a Microsurgical Femoral Vein Access. *J. Reconstr. Microsurg.* **2015**, *31*, 343–347. [CrossRef] [PubMed]

94. Gaines Das, R.; North, D. Implications of experimental technique for analysis and interpretation of data from animal experiments: Outliers and increased variability resulting from failure of intraperitoneal injection procedures. *Lab. Anim.* **2007**, *41*, 312–320. [CrossRef] [PubMed]
95. Laferriere, C.A.; Pang, D.S. Review of Intraperitoneal Injection of Sodium Pentobarbital as a Method of Euthanasia in Laboratory Rodents. *J. Am. Assoc. Lab. Anim. Sci.* **2020**, *59*, 254–263. [CrossRef]
96. Gargiulo, S.; Greco, A.; Gramanzini, M.; Esposito, S.; Affuso, A.; Brunetti, A.; Vesce, G. Mice anesthesia, analgesia, and care, Part I: Anesthetic considerations in preclinical research. *Ilar. J.* **2012**, *53*, E55–E69. [CrossRef]
97. Smiler, K.L.; Stein, S.; Hrapkiewicz, K.L.; Hiben, J.R. Tissue response to intramuscular and intraperitoneal injections of ketamine and xylazine in rats. *Lab. Anim. Sci.* **1990**, *40*, 60–64.
98. Vogler, G.A. Chapter 5—Anesthesia Delivery Systems. In *Anesthesia and Analgesia in Laboratory Animals*, 2nd ed.; Fish, R.E., Brown, M.J., Danneman, P.J., Karas, A.Z., Eds.; Academic Press: San Diego, CA, USA, 2008; pp. 127–169.
99. Obernier, J.A.; Baldwin, R.L. Establishing an appropriate period of acclimatization following transportation of laboratory animals. *Ilar. J.* **2006**, *47*, 364–369. [CrossRef]
100. Milligan, S.R.; Sales, G.D.; Khirnykh, K. Sound levels in rooms housing laboratory animals: An uncontrolled daily variable. *Physiol. Behav.* **1993**, *53*, 1067–1076. [CrossRef]
101. Lauer, A.M.; Larkin, G.; Jones, A.; May, B.J. Behavioral Animal Model of the Emotional Response to Tinnitus and Hearing Loss. *J. Assoc. Res. Otolaryngol.* **2018**, *19*, 67–81. [CrossRef] [PubMed]
102. Gouveia, K.; Hurst, J.L. Optimising reliability of mouse performance in behavioural testing: The major role of non-aversive handling. *Sci. Rep.* **2017**, *7*, 44999. [CrossRef] [PubMed]
103. Georgiou, P.; Zanos, P.; Mou, T.M.; An, X.; Gerhard, D.M.; Dryanovski, D.I.; Potter, L.E.; Highland, J.N.; Jenne, C.E.; Stewart, B.W.; et al. Experimenters' sex modulates mouse behaviors and neural responses to ketamine via corticotropin releasing factor. *Nat. Neurosci.* **2022**, *25*, 1191–1200. [CrossRef]
104. Van Driel, K.S.; Talling, J.C. Familiarity increases consistency in animal tests. *Behav. Brain Res.* **2005**, *159*, 243–245. [CrossRef]
105. Theilmann, W.; Kleimann, A.; Rhein, M.; Bleich, S.; Frieling, H.; Löscher, W.; Brandt, C. Behavioral differences of male Wistar rats from different vendors in vulnerability and resilience to chronic mild stress are reflected in epigenetic regulation and expression of p11. *Brain Res.* **2016**, *1642*, 505–515. [CrossRef] [PubMed]
106. Castelhano-Carlos, M.J.; Baumans, V. The impact of light, noise, cage cleaning and in-house transport on welfare and stress of laboratory rats. *Lab. Anim.* **2009**, *43*, 311–327. [CrossRef]
107. Pérez-Valenzuela, C.; Gárate-Pérez, M.F.; Sotomayor-Zárate, R.; Delano, P.H.; Dagnino-Subiabre, A. Reboxetine Improves Auditory Attention and Increases Norepinephrine Levels in the Auditory Cortex of Chronically Stressed Rats. *Front. Neural Circuits* **2016**, *10*, 108. [CrossRef]
108. Karp, N.A.; Pearl, E.J.; Stringer, E.J.; Barkus, C.; Ulrichsen, J.C.; Percie du Sert, N. A qualitative study of the barriers to using blinding in in vivo experiments and suggestions for improvement. *PLoS Biol.* **2022**, *20*, e3001873. [CrossRef]
109. Schrode, K.M.; Dent, M.L.; Lauer, A.M. Sources of variability in auditory brainstem response thresholds in a mouse model of noise-induced hearing loss. *J. Acoust. Soc. Am.* **2022**, *152*, 3576. [CrossRef]
110. Available online: https://www.tdt.com/docs/abr-user-guide/troubleshooting/#determining-the-noise-floor (accessed on 15 April 2023).
111. Van Eenige, R.; Verhave, P.S.; Koemans, P.J.; Tiebosch, I.; Rensen, P.C.N.; Kooijman, S. RandoMice, a novel, user-friendly randomization tool in animal research. *PLoS ONE* **2020**, *15*, e0237096. [CrossRef]
112. Available online: https://www.gv-solas.de/wp-content/uploads/2021/08/2020_10Food_withdrawal.pdf (accessed on 24 March 2023).
113. Varughese, S.; Ahmed, R. Environmental and Occupational Considerations of Anesthesia: A Narrative Review and Update. *Anesth. Analg.* **2021**, *133*, 826–835. [CrossRef] [PubMed]
114. Akil, O.; Oursler, A.E.; Fan, K.; Lustig, L.R. Mouse Auditory Brainstem Response Testing. *Bio Protoc.* **2016**, *6*, 1–7. [CrossRef] [PubMed]
115. Navarro, K.L.; Huss, M.; Smith, J.C.; Sharp, P.; Marx, J.O.; Pacharinsak, C. Mouse Anesthesia: The Art and Science. *Ilar. J.* **2021**, *62*, 238–273. [CrossRef] [PubMed]
116. Rossi, G.T.; Britt, R.H. Effects of hypothermia on the cat brain-stem auditory evoked response. *Electroencephalogr. Clin. Neurophysiol.* **1984**, *57*, 143–155. [CrossRef]
117. Jones, T.A.; Stockard, J.J.; Weidner, W.J. The effects of temperature and acute alcohol intoxication on brain stem auditory evoked potentials in the cat. *Electroencephalogr. Clin. Neurophysiol.* **1980**, *49*, 23–30. [CrossRef]
118. Terkildsen, K.; Osterhammel, P. The influence of reference electrode position on recordings of the auditory brainstem responses. *Ear Hear.* **1981**, *2*, 9–14. [CrossRef]
119. Manta, O.; Sarafidis, M.; Vasileiou, N.; Schlee, W.; Consoulas, C.; Kikidis, D.; Vassou, E.; Matsopoulos, G.K.; Koutsouris, D.D. Development and Evaluation of Automated Tools for Auditory-Brainstem and Middle-Auditory Evoked Potentials Waves Detection and Annotation. *Brain Sci.* **2022**, *12*, 1675. [CrossRef]
120. Bogaerts, S.; Clements, J.D.; Sullivan, J.M.; Oleskevich, S. Automated threshold detection for auditory brainstem responses: Comparison with visual estimation in a stem cell transplantation study. *BMC Neurosci.* **2009**, *10*, 104. [CrossRef]

121. Teixeira da Silva, J.A. Room temperature in scientific protocols and experiments should be defined: A reproducibility issue. *Biotechniques* **2021**, *70*, 306–308. [CrossRef]
122. Willott, J.F. Measurement of the auditory brainstem response (ABR) to study auditory sensitivity in mice. *Curr. Protoc. Neurosci.* **2006**, *Chapter 8*, Unit8.21B. [CrossRef]
123. Ingham, N.J.; Pearson, S.; Steel, K.P. Using the Auditory Brainstem Response (ABR) to Determine Sensitivity of Hearing in Mutant Mice. *Curr. Protoc. Mouse Biol.* **2011**, *1*, 279–287. [CrossRef] [PubMed]
124. Zeng, L.; Zhou, W.; Bing, D.; Xie, L.; Wang, X.; Zhang, G. Protocol for assessing auditory brainstem response in mice using a four-channel recording system. *STAR Protoc.* **2022**, *3*, 101251. [CrossRef] [PubMed]
125. Percie du Sert, N.; Hurst, V.; Ahluwalia, A.; Alam, S.; Avey, M.T.; Baker, M.; Browne, W.J.; Clark, A.; Cuthill, I.C.; Dirnagl, U.; et al. The ARRIVE guidelines 2.0: Updated guidelines for reporting animal research. *PLoS Biol.* **2020**, *18*, e3000410. [CrossRef]
126. Scudamore, C.L.; Soilleux, E.J.; Karp, N.A.; Smith, K.; Poulsom, R.; Herrington, C.S.; Day, M.J.; Brayton, C.F.; Bolon, B.; Whitelaw, B.; et al. Recommendations for minimum information for publication of experimental pathology data: MINPEPA guidelines. *J. Pathol.* **2016**, *238*, 359–367. [CrossRef] [PubMed]

Disclaimer/Publisher's Note: The statements, opinions and data contained in all publications are solely those of the individual author(s) and contributor(s) and not of MDPI and/or the editor(s). MDPI and/or the editor(s) disclaim responsibility for any injury to people or property resulting from any ideas, methods, instructions or products referred to in the content.

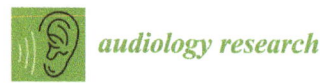

Article

The Effect of Pluronic-Coated Gold Nanoparticles in Hearing Preservation Following Cochlear Implantation-Pilot Study

Cristina Maria Blebea [1], Violeta Necula [1,2], Monica Potara [3], Maximilian George Dindelegan [1], Laszlo Peter Ujvary [1,*], Emil Claudiu Botan [4], Alma Aurelia Maniu [1,2] and Marcel Cosgarea [1]

1. Department of Otorhinolaryngology, "Iuliu Hatieganu" University of Medicine and Pharmacy, 400337 Cluj-Napoca, Romania
2. Department of Otolaryngology, Emergency County Hospital, 400006 Cluj-Napoca, Romania
3. Nanobiophotonics and Laser Microspectroscopy Center, Interdisciplinary Research Institute in Bio-Nano-Sciences, Babes-Bolyai University, T. Laurian Str. 42, 400271 Cluj-Napoca, Romania
4. Department of Pathology, Emergency County Hospital, 400337 Cluj-Napoca, Romania
* Correspondence: ujvarypeter@outlook.com; Tel.: +40-746403264

Citation: Blebea, C.M.; Necula, V.; Potara, M.; Dindelegan, M.G.; Ujvary, L.P.; Botan, E.C.; Maniu, A.A.; Cosgarea, M. The Effect of Pluronic-Coated Gold Nanoparticles in Hearing Preservation Following Cochlear Implantation-Pilot Study. *Audiol. Res.* **2022**, *12*, 466–475. https://doi.org/10.3390/audiolres12050047

Academic Editor: Agnieszka Szczepek

Received: 26 July 2022
Accepted: 24 August 2022
Published: 28 August 2022

Publisher's Note: MDPI stays neutral with regard to jurisdictional claims in published maps and institutional affiliations.

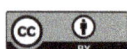

Copyright: © 2022 by the authors. Licensee MDPI, Basel, Switzerland. This article is an open access article distributed under the terms and conditions of the Creative Commons Attribution (CC BY) license (https://creativecommons.org/licenses/by/4.0/).

Abstract: Introduction: During cochlear implantation, electrode insertion can cause cochlear damage, inflammation, and apoptosis, which can affect the residual hearing. Nanoparticles are increasingly studied as a way to increase the availability of inner ear protective factors. We studied the effect on rats of Pluronic-coated gold nanoparticles (Plu-AuNPs) containing dexamethasone, which were applied locally in the rat's middle ear following the implant procedure. Methods: Seven rats were used in the study. The right ear served as a model for the Dex-Plu-AuNP group. Following the intracochlear dummy electrode insertion through the round window, Dex-Plu-AuNPs were placed in the round window niche. In the right ear, following the same insertion procedure, free dexamethasone (Dex) was placed in the same manner. Auditory brainstem response thresholds (click stimulus, pure tones at 8 kHz, 16 kHz, 24 kHz, and 32 kHz) were measured before and one week after the procedure. A two-tailed T-test was used for the variables. Statistical significance was set as $p < 0.05$. Results: In the Dex-Plu-AuNP group, the threshold shift was less than that in the free dexamethasone group, but no statistical significance was noted between the groups. When compared individually, only the 8 kHz frequency showed statistically significant, better results after one week, in favor of the Dex-Plu-AuNP group. The mean postoperative 8 kHz threshold in the Dex-Plu-AuNPs was significantly lower than that of the control group ($p = 0.048$, t-test). For the other frequencies, statistical analysis showed no significant differences between the mean threshold shifts of the two cohorts. Conclusions: The local application of Plu-AuNPs containing dexamethasone following cochlear implantation may better protect the residual hearing than dexamethasone alone, but a larger sample size is needed to reach a possible statistical significance. Dex-Plu-AuNPs do not seem to cause ototoxicity and may be used as a carrier for other agents. In a clinical setting, Dex-Plu-AuNPs may have the effect of protecting lower frequencies in patients with partial deafness who are candidates for electric acoustic stimulation (EAS). If we consider this tendency, Dex-Plu-AuNPs may also be beneficial for patients with Ménière's disease.

Keywords: hearing loss; cochlear implant; nanomaterials; ABR; Pluronic; dexamethasone

1. Introduction

Reducing cochlear damage and preserving the residual hearing capacity has long been a primary objective of inner ear procedures, particularly cochlear implantation (CI) [1]. In recent years, growing interest can be observed regarding hearing conservation in candidates for hybrid, electro-acoustic stimulation whose residual hearing levels may be affected during CI [2,3]. As patients with partial deafness (PD) can benefit from a CI, members of the HEARRING group have extensively studied hearing preservation in cochlear implantation (HPCI) in adults and children, using a variety of electrode array types and manufacturers [4,5]. Limiting the cochlear trauma during CI is also beneficial for patients with minimal residual hearing as larger amounts of electrically induced information passing through a healthier neural interface will promote better speech discrimination [6].

The loss of hearing remnants following CI surgery, especially for low frequencies, generally presents two possible outcomes: an early and a late phase. The immediate loss of residual hearing can be due to insertion trauma (fracture of the osseous spiral lamina, displacement of the basilar membrane, damage to the stria vascularis, or disturbance of the cochlear fluids) and the subsequent inflammatory response [1]. Later residual hearing loss can occur months after implantation. Such a loss can be progressive, fluctuating, or sudden, and its identification largely depends on the observation period and the frequency of visits to the audiologist [7]. Most of the available information regarding the cochlear inflammatory response and its modulation has been gathered through experimental models; scarce data is available from human postmortem studies.

The prospects of HPCI have greatly increased with the development of less traumatic electrodes, in conjunction with the application of soft surgery principles [8]. As surgical principles and electrode design have been extensively studied, attention is shifting toward new solutions, such as assisted electrode insertion or otoprotective pharmacological support through either systemic or local drug delivery [1]. Local drug delivery using novel nanoparticles (NPs) via the intratympanic or intracochlear route is intended to generate high localized concentrations while avoiding any systemic side effects.

Metallic and metal oxide nanoparticles are among the most promising inorganic substances for the treatment of inner ear diseases [9]. Gold nanoparticles (AuNPs) are distinguished by their superior chemical and physical stability. They can be functionalized with organic molecules that are biologically active, granting them excellent biocompatibility, and can be used for loading drugs or as inner ear contrast agents [10,11].

NP-based medication delivery can be employed to reduce inflammation and fibrosis after CI and to maintain residual hearing. In recent years, the number of FDA approvals for the use of NPs to treat various auditory diseases has increased [11]. In a preclinical setting, locally applied chitosan-coated gold nanoparticles (Cs-AuNPs) in the rats' tympanic bulla did not compromise the animals' hearing thresholds [12]. However, AuNPs have not yet been utilized in treating inner ear diseases. Other types of AuNPs, like pluronic-coated Au-NPs, seem to have promising results regarding drug distribution and hemocompatibility [13]. The current experimental pilot study aims to evaluate if Pluronic-coated AuNPs carrying dexamethasone (Dex-Plu-AuNPs) can yield better auditory brainstem response (ABR) thresholds, compared to free dexamethasone (Dex), and if they can better protect against the progressive cochlear function loss developed following electrode insertion trauma.

2. Materials and Methods

2.1. Animals

Seven adult male Wistar rats, weighing 250–300 g, with good general health were included in a prospective randomized experimental pilot study. Otologic inclusion criteria were considered to be good general health and the absence of otitis media. All the included subjects were endoscopically screened to exclude external and middle ear pathology. All protocols were conducted according to European law regarding the welfare of experimental animals and followed the guidelines established by our institution's ethical committee (AVZ 81/28.03.2022) and the National Veterinary Health and Food Safety Authority (ethical approval no. 316/30.05.2022). Following the 3Rs approach [14], we minimized the number of subjects by using both ears of each subject to compare the two forms of dexamethasone delivery.

2.2. Chemicals

Trisodium citrate ($C_6H_5Na_3O_7 \cdot 2H_2O$, $\geq$99%), hydrogen tetrachloroaurate (III) hydrate ($HAuCl_4 \cdot 3H_2O$, 99.99%), Pluronic F127, and dexamethasone were purchased from

Sigma-Aldrich. Ethanol (96%) was obtained from Chemical Company, Iași, Romania. All chemicals were used without further purification. The aqueous solutions were prepared using ultrapure water.

2.3. Nanoparticles Preparation and Loading with Dexamethasone

Citrate-capped gold nanoparticles (AuNPs) of spherical shape were prepared according to the Turkevich–Frens method [15]. In brief, 100 mL of an aqueous solution of $HAuCl_4 \cdot 3H_2O$ (10^{-3} M) was boiled on a magnetic stirring hot plate. Then, 10 mL of an aqueous sodium citrate solution (38.8×10^{-3} M) was quickly added while maintaining magnetic stirring. The stirring process was continued for 10–15 min after the color of the colloidal suspension became a deep burgundy red. The color changes in the solution from yellow to intense burgundy red indicate the formation of colloidal nanoparticles. Pluronic-coated gold nanoparticles (Plu-AuNPs) were obtained by incubating AuNPs with an aqueous Pluronic F127 solution at a final concentration of 4×10^{-4} M. The obtained Plu-AuNP suspension was then purified by centrifugation at 12,000 rpm for 20 min. To prepare dexamethasone-loaded Plu-AuNPs (Dex-Plu-AuNPs), the colloidal solution was incubated with Dex at a final concentration of 0.18 mg/mL, and the resulting mixture was ultrasonicated for 50 min. The prepared Dex-AuNP nanoconjugate was then incubated with Pluronic F127 (4×10^{-4} M), followed by centrifugation to remove the unbound polymer and drug. The formation of Dex-Plu-AuNPs was monitored by UV–visible absorption spectroscopy, using a Jasco V-670 UV–vis-NIR spectrometer (JASCO, Hachioji, Tokyo, Japan). The concentration of loaded Dex was estimated indirectly, according to the Beer–Lambert law, by calculating the amount of unloaded Dex molecules remaining in the supernatant. The final concentration of loaded Dex was 10 μg/mL. The concentration of gold nanoparticles expressed in μg/mL was determined by atomic absorption spectroscopy (Avanta PM, GBC-Australia (GBC Scientific Equipment, Braeside, Victoria, Australia)).

2.4. Anesthesia, Surgical Preparation, and Approach

Anesthesia was achieved using a mix of Ketamine (80 mg/kg) and Xylazine (8 mg/kg), administered intramuscularly [16]. Additional doses were administered during the procedure if signs of pain were observed (withdrawal reflex to a plantar pinch or eyelid reflex). During the procedure, the animal was kept at a constant body temperature of 35–37 °C using a heating pad, and the eyes were protected from drying using a sterile ophthalmic solution. Animals recovered post-operatively in separate cages, with free access to water and food.

The surgical intervention was performed using a Leica® microscope (Model M320, Leica, Wetzlar, Hesse, Germany). Insertion of the electrode analog was achieved via the round window (RW), using a retroauricular approach to the tympanic bulla. Access to the middle ear was achieved through a bony defect in the posteroinferior aspect of the bulla. A 1-millimeter diameter cutting drill was used to access the bony defect, with good exposure of the stapedial artery, RW niche, and RW membrane (Figure 1). The bony defect of the middle ear was sealed using the surrounding muscles. Finally, the platysmal muscle and skin were sutured with absorbable Vicryl 6/0 sutures (Ethicon®, Raritan, NJ, USA). The wound was covered with a topical spray containing oxytetracycline. All surgical procedures were performed under aseptic conditions.

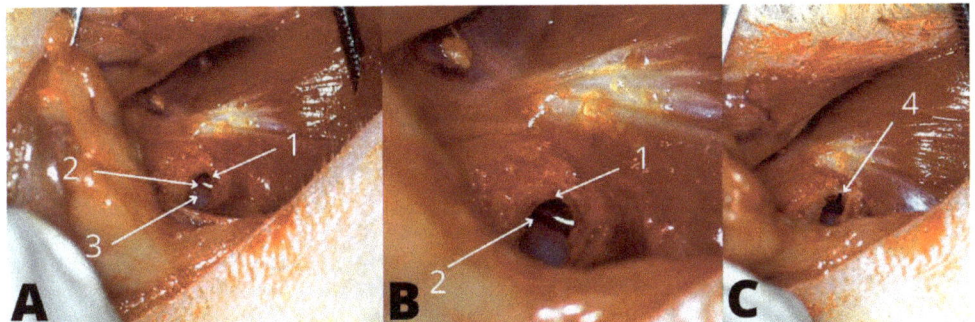

Figure 1. Left ear electrode analog insertion; 1—round window niche; 2—stapedial artery; 3—middle ear, seen through the bony defect; 4—electrode analog during the insertion through the round window membrane. (**A**): Opening of the left middle ear, (**B**): Visualization of the RW, (**C**): Left ear electrode analog insertion.

2.5. Dummy Electrode

A monofilament 5/0 polypropylene suture (Ethicon®, Raritan, NJ, USA) with a length of 5 mm was employed for the insertion [17,18].

2.6. Groups

To reduce the number of animals included in the study, we divided the groups as follows. One ear was considered to represent the study group (group 1) with the contralateral ear representing the control group (group 2). In group 1, after inserting the analog electrode through the RW, 30 µL of Dex-Plu-AuNP solution was applied in the middle ear and above the RW. The concentration of Plu-AuNPs was 1005 µg/mL, while the dexamethasone concentration was 64 µg/mL. In group 2, after the same insertion procedure, 30 µL of free Dex solution with a dexamethasone concentration of 64 µg/mL was applied.

2.7. Hearing Threshold Measurement: Auditory Brainstem Response (ABR)

All rats included in the study presented normal hearing before surgery. We determined the hearing thresholds bilaterally before surgery and seven days following the implantation procedure. We assessed the external and middle ear status before the audiological measurements, to exclude a conductive hearing loss component.

We measured ABR thresholds in a soundproof room using the Opti-Amp bio amplifier (Intelligent Hearing System, Miami, FL, USA) connected to the Smart EP system. Click stimulus, and pure tones of 8 kHz, 16 kHz, 24 kHz, and 32 kHz were presented through closed tubes placed into the external ear canal, with 1.3 ms duration at a 20/s repetition rate. ER insert earphones were used for the click stimulus and high-frequency transducers were used for the tone burst stimulus. Stainless steel needle electrodes were placed subcutaneously in the retroauricular area (recording negative electrode), on the vertex (positive reference), and rear leg (ground electrode). Ipsilateral evoked potentials were averaged over 1024 sweeps in decreasing intensity increments of 10 dB SPL; thresholds were defined as the minimum stimulating level with an ABR response that can be identifiable and repeatable.

2.8. Statistics

IBM® SPSS® (IBM, Armonk, NY, USA) was used for statistical analysis. Analyses were performed on the outcome measures between pre-implantation (T0) and post-implantation (T1). A two-tailed Student's *t*-test was used for independent variables to assess group heterogeneity, as well as to compare pre- and post-implantation audiological data, represented as dB SPL for the selected frequencies. The significance level was set at $p < 0.05$.

3. Results

3.1. Spectral Characterization of Dex-Plu-AuNPs

Figure 2A illustrates the normalized UV-Vis absorption spectra of AuNPs before and after stabilization with Pluronic F127. As one can observe, citrate-capped AuNPs exhibit a plasmonic band with an extinction maximum at 519 nm, which represents the typical spectral signature of spherical colloidal gold nanoparticles. Stabilization with Pluronic induced a 2 nm shift toward higher wavelengths, due to the modification of the refractive index of the surrounding medium. Normalized UV-Vis absorption spectra before and after Dex loading are depicted in Figure 2B, taken after each preparation step. The inset of Figure 2B illustrates the magnified spectral region of the absorption maxima. We noticed that the spectra of Dex-AuNPs and Dex-Plu-AuNPs showed a hybrid profile containing both the spectral signature of AuNPs and the electronic absorption of Dex molecules in the UV spectral domain at 240 nm. Moreover, the plasmonic band of Dex-AuNPs experiences a 2 nm red shift compared to AuNPs, followed by a further 2 nm shift toward higher wavelengths upon stabilization with Pluronic.

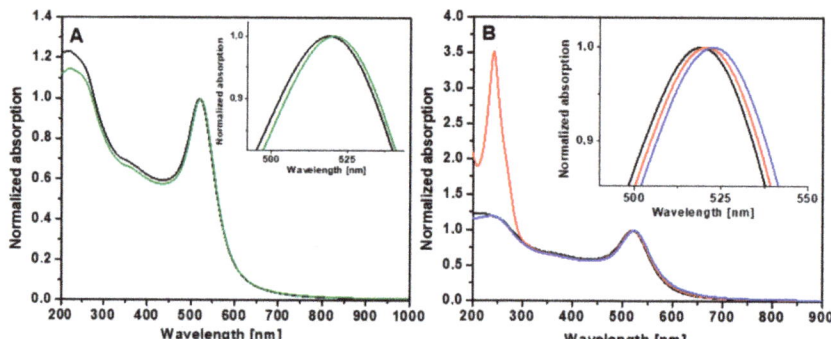

Figure 2. (**A**) Normalized UV-Vis absorption spectra of AuNPs (black) and Plu-AuNPs (green). (**B**) Normalized UV-Vis absorption spectra of AuNPs (black), Dex-AuNPs (red), and Plu-Dex-AuNPs (blue). The inserts show the magnified spectral region of the absorption maxima.

These spectral changes are related to the modification of the refractive index of the medium surrounding the particles due to the attachment of Dex onto the gold surface and encapsulation with Pluronic F127.

3.2. Audiological Results

Before cochlear implantation, all rats presented similar hearing thresholds in both ears (Table 1). There was no statistical difference between the median values of the hearing threshold at any of the used stimuli (p values > 0.05, *t*-test).

Table 1. Preoperative frequency-specific hearing threshold (dB SPL) for both the Dex-Plu-AuNP and Dex groups.

Stimuli	Dex-Plu-AuNPs (*n* = 7)		Dex (*n* = 7)		*p* Value (*t*-Test)
	Threshold Mean (dB SPL)	SD	Threshold Mean (dB SPL)	SD	
Click	20	0	20	0	-
8 kHz	20	0	20.7	1.8	0.35
16 kHz	20	0	20.7	1.8	0.35
24 kHz	20	0	20	0	-
32 kHz	21.4	10.6	22.85	5.6	0.59

The two-tailed *t*-test indicates no significant difference between groups ($p > 0.05$); SD = standard deviation; dB SPL = decibel sound pressure level; kHz = kilohertz; n = number of subjects.

One week after implantation, neither animal displayed otorrhea, signs of middle ear infection, or infection at the incision site. Therefore, the determinations of ABR thresholds followed the same protocol as the preoperative ones.

At seven days after bilateral CI, both groups displayed a significant elevation in hearing threshold across all frequency ranges (Table 2). When individual frequencies were analyzed one week after surgery, the Dex-Plu-AuNP group averaged better hearing thresholds than the dexamethasone group. However, no statistical significance was noted between the two groups, except for one frequency.

Table 2. Postoperative frequency-specific hearing threshold (SPL dB) for both the Dex-Plu-AuNP and Dex cohorts.

Stimuli	Group	N	Mean dB SPL	Std. Deviation	Std. Error Mean
clickpost	Dex-Plu-AuNPs	7	63.57	28.536	10.785
	Dex	7	74.29	21.876	8.268
post8 kHz	Dex-Plu-AuNPs	7	87.86	23.954	9.054
	Dex	7	108.57	6.901	2.608
post16 kHz	Dex-Plu-AuNPs	7	97.14	18.225	6.888
	Dex	7	108.57	14.351	5.424
post24 kHz	Dex-Plu-AuNPs	7	70.71	16.439	6.213
	Dex	7	79.29	14.840	5.609
post32 kHz	Dex-Plu-AuNPs	7	87.14	11.852	4.480
	Dex	7	92.86	10.746	4.062

Dex-Plu-AuNPs = Pluronic-coated gold nanoparticles with dexamethasone; Dex = free form of dexamethasone; dB SPL = decibel sound pressure level; kHz = kilohertz; post = postoperative.

At 8 kHz, there was a significant difference of 20.7 dB between the mean thresholds of the two groups in favor of the Dex-Plu-AuNP group (Dex = 108.57, Dex-Plu-AuNP = 87.86, $p = 0.048$, *t*-test) (Figure 2).

At 16 kHz, there was a statistically insignificant difference of 11.43 dB between the mean threshold of the two groups in favor of the Dex-Plu-AuNP group (Dex = 108.57 dB, Dex-Plu-AuNPs = 97.14 dB, $p = 0.21$, *t*-test) (Figure 3). At 24 kHz, the difference between the mean threshold of the two cohorts was 8.5 dB; however, this difference did not reach significance (Dex = 79.29, Dex-Plu-AuNPs = 70.71, $p = 0.32$) (Figure 3). In addition, the highest frequency, recorded at 32 kHz, did not yield any significant difference between the groups at 5.7 dB (Dex = 92.86, Dex-Plu-AuNPs = 87.14, $p = 0.36$, *t*-test) (Figure 3).

The click stimulus elicited the least amount of threshold shift in the control and study groups, with a difference of 10.7 dB between them. However, the difference was not statistically significant (Dex = 74.29, Dex-Plu-AuNPs = 63.57, $p = 0.44$, *t*-test) (Figure 4).

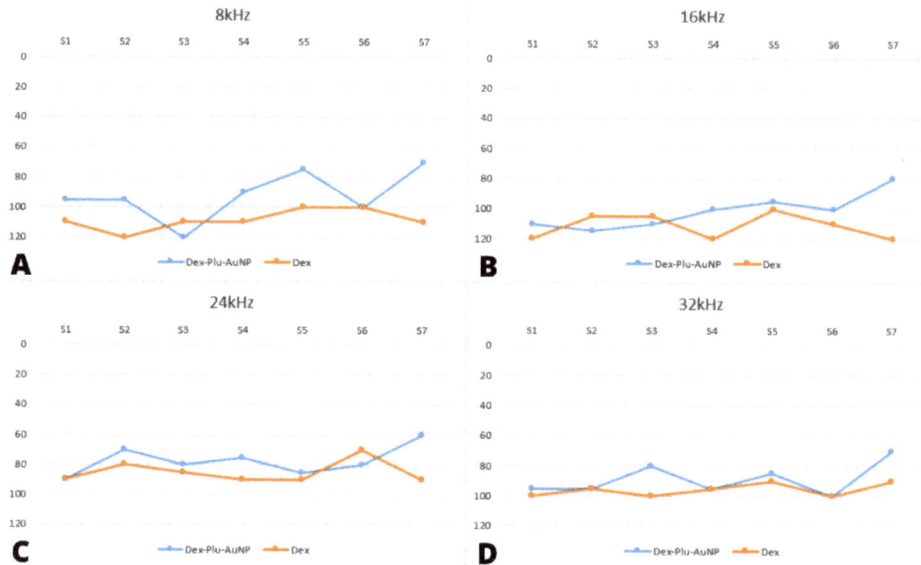

Figure 3. Representation of postoperative hearing threshold for rats in both groups, measured through auditory brainstem response. Results are presented as individual values for each subject at a specific frequency. (**A**) 8 kHz; (**B**) 16 kHz; (**C**) 24 kHz; (**D**) 32 kHz; dB SPL = sound pressure level expressed in decibels; Dex-Plu-AuNP= Pluronic-coated gold nanoparticles with dexamethasone; Dex = free form of dexamethasone; kHz = kilohertz; S = subject.

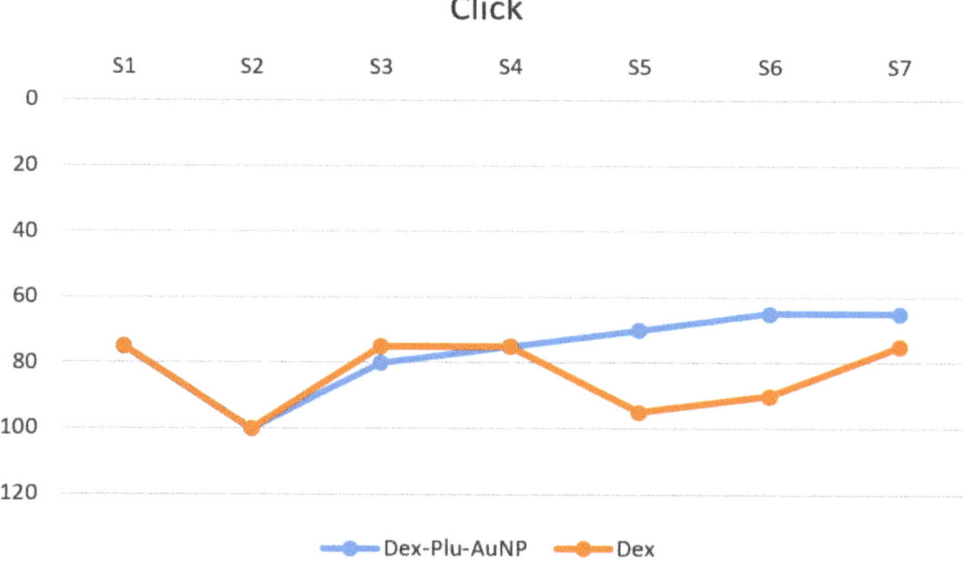

Figure 4. Postoperative hearing threshold using click stimuli; dB SPL = sound pressure level expressed in decibels; Dex-Plu-AuNPs = Pluronic-coated gold nanoparticles with dexamethasone; Dex = free form of dexamethasone; kHz = kilohertz; S = subject.

4. Discussion

Since cochlear surgery can be considered a traumatic event, it is of the utmost importance to maintain the normal architecture and surface anatomy throughout the early periods of recuperation. The reduction of local trauma and preservation of long-term residual hearing are major focuses for patients undergoing cochlear implantation surgery. There have been many attempts to develop adjuvant therapy strategies to avoid or diminish the acute and late inflammatory phases seen after CI. Corticosteroid usage had a substantial influence on auditory brainstem response, impedance, and histopathological alterations in the animal models. However, the otoprotective effect was only long-lasting with continued administration [19,20]. Clinical trials fail to provide consistent recommendations regarding the routes of administration as well as dosage [21–24]. The cost of hospitalization for intravenous corticosteroid administration and the possible side effects of systemic administration open up the possibility of researching methods of local delivery. To render efficiency and prolong the local effect of corticosteroids, different strategies have been addressed, one of them being the usage of nanocarriers.

AuNPs belong to a promising nanocarrier-mediated drug delivery class; they have easy surface functionalization and the ability to modify their size, shape, and surface chemistry [11]. They also exhibit ROS-independent antimicrobial activity, making them safer for mammalian cells than the other nanometals [25]. Using AuNPs as an intratympanic vector can allow patients to benefit from these characteristics. Nevertheless, the possible variations of these parameters make it hard to truly study their toxicity. Initial in vivo studies researching their utility as an inner ear contrast agent observed no effect on the morphology of the hair cells [12,26].

The results of this study confirm some of the previous observations regarding the significant and variable nature of hearing loss after cochlear implantation in experimental models [27]. The limitations of this study would be the reduced number of subjects included. In addition, the nature of the surgical procedure itself can be subject to human variation and needs to be considered a variable.

Our study's hearing threshold shift was greater than other rodent-based CI experimental models [18]. Although the threshold shift values we obtained in the study were high, another study using the same length (5 mm) of electrode analog also reported high hearing threshold shifts of approximately 65 ± 27 dB [17]. Even though these values are higher than the literature reports, they are consistent throughout all the subjects of both groups; therefore, the repeatability of the surgical maneuvers can be considered to have been accomplished. The full-length insertion of the dummy electrode and its material can be a possible source for the obtained results. The otoendoscopic evaluation eliminated the possibility of middle ear conduction interference that could have influenced the results.

The results that have emerged from our study show the tendency for a lower hearing threshold shift in the group where CI was associated with Dex-Plu-AuNPs, but no statistical difference was noted except at the 8 kHz frequency. Obtaining better protection of the lower frequencies is the desired effect when considering CI in patients with residual hearing. A larger study group could elicit further information about the sustainability of this finding.

On the other hand, when considering the possible cell toxicity, if no statistical significance was noted between the two groups, it is plausible to add that Plu-AuNPs presented no ototoxicity in the short term. Therefore, this carrier can be considered a safe alternative delivery method for other possible otoprotective agents. In the future, we need to pursue more extended follow-up periods through audiological threshold measures and note histopathological alterations considering different Dex and Plu-AuNP concentrations.

Translating the effect of Dex-Plu-AuNPs in a clinical setting may serve as a better alternative to utilizing free Dex, offering beneficial preventive short-term residual hearing protection from damage caused by the cochlear implantation process itself. The short-term effects do not suggest any cytotoxicity but rather imply a protective effect on hearing thresholds. The potential to better protect lower frequencies needs to be further studied; cochlear implant recommendations have expanded to include patients with partial deafness who are candidates for electric acoustic stimulation (EAS). Clinical implementation can be also beneficial for patients with Ménière's disease, in which the low frequencies are initially those most affected.

5. Conclusions

Pluronic-coated AuNPs carrying dexamethasone, applied to the round window, may be useful as an additional treatment for limiting the short-term inner-ear damage caused by cochlear implantation, along with the soft surgery principles. The long-term effects need to be evaluated, together with the capacity to sustain a delayed and prolonged anti-inflammatory effect. Since no statistical differences were found in the audiological parameters, more evidence is needed to support the use of Plu-AuNPs containing dexamethasone as a pharmacological compound for the protection of residual hearing. Dexamethasone may be beneficial in its free form without the need for a carrier.

Author Contributions: Conceptualization, C.M.B., A.A.M. and M.C.; methodology, C.M.B., M.P. and M.G.D.; validation, M.C., A.A.M. and V.N.; investigation, C.M.B., M.G.D., L.P.U. and E.C.B.; data curation, L.P.U. and V.N.; writing—original draft preparation, C.M.B. and L.P.U.; writing—review and editing, L.P.U., C.M.B. and A.A.M.; visualization, V.N.; supervision, M.C. and A.A.M.; funding acquisition, A.A.M. All authors have read and agreed to the published version of the manuscript.

Funding: This work was supported by the CNCS-UEFISCDI, project number PN-III-P2-2.1-PED-2019-381.

Institutional Review Board Statement: All protocols were conducted according to European law and welfare of experimental animals and followed the guidelines established by our institution's ethical committee (AVZ 81/28.03.2022) and the National Veterinary Health and Food Safety Authority (ethical approval no. 316/30.05.2022).

Informed Consent Statement: Not applicable.

Data Availability Statement: The data presented in this study are available on request from the corresponding author.

Conflicts of Interest: The authors declare no conflict of interest.

References

1. Blebea, C.M.; Ujvary, L.P.; Necula, V.; Dindelegan, M.G.; Perde-Schrepler, M.; Stamate, M.C.; Cosgarea, M.; Maniu, A.A. Current Concepts and Future Trends in Increasing the Benefits of Cochlear Implantation: A Narrative Review. *Medicina* **2022**, *58*, 747. [CrossRef]
2. Park, L.R.; Teagle, H.F.B.; Gagnon, E.; Woodard, J.; Brown, K.D. Electric-Acoustic Stimulation Outcomes in Children. *Ear Hear.* **2019**, *40*, 849–857. [CrossRef]
3. Rader, T.; Bohnert, A.; Matthias, C.; Koutsimpelas, D.; Kainz, M.A.; Strieth, S. Hearing Preservation in Children with Electric-Acoustic Stimulation after Cochlear Implantation: Outcome after Electrode Insertion with Minimal Insertion Trauma. *HNO* **2018**, *66*, 56–62. [CrossRef]
4. Rajan, G.; Tavora-Vieira, D.; Baumgartner, W.D.; Godey, B.; Müller, J.; O'Driscoll, M.; Skarzynski, H.; Skarzynski, P.; Usami, S.I.; Adunka, O.; et al. Hearing Preservation Cochlear Implantation in Children: The HEARRING Group Consensus and Practice Guide. *Cochlear Implant. Int.* **2017**, *19*, 1–13. [CrossRef]
5. Matin, F.; Artukarslan, E.N.; Illg, A.; Lesinski-Schiedat, A.; Lenarz, T.; Suhling, M.C. Cochlear Implantation in Elderly Patients with Residual Hearing. *J. Clin. Med.* **2021**, *10*, 4305. [CrossRef]
6. Skarzynski, H.; Van De Heyning, P.; Agrawal, S.; Arauz, S.L.; Atlas, M.; Baumgartner, W.; Caversaccio, M.; De Bodt, M.; Gavilan, J.; Godey, B.; et al. Towards a Consensus on a Hearing Preservation Classification System. *Acta Oto-Laryngol.* **2013**, *133*, 3–13. [CrossRef] [PubMed]
7. Foggia, M.J.; Quevedo, R.V.; Hansen, M.R. Intracochlear Fibrosis and the Foreign Body Response to Cochlear Implant Biomaterials. *Laryngoscope Investig. Otolaryngol.* **2019**, *4*, 678–683. [CrossRef] [PubMed]
8. Khater, A.; El-Anwar, M.W. Methods of Hearing Preservation during Cochlear Implantation. *Int. Arch. Otorhinolaryngol.* **2017**, *21*, 297–301. [CrossRef] [PubMed]
9. Xu, X.; Zheng, J.; He, Y.; Lin, K.; Li, S.; Zhang, Y.; Song, P.; Zhou, Y.; Chen, X. Nanocarriers for Inner Ear Disease Therapy. *Front. Cell. Neurosci.* **2021**, *15*, 791573. [CrossRef] [PubMed]
10. Dindelegan, M.G.; Blebea, C.; Perde-Schrepler, M.; Buzoianu, A.D.; Maniu, A.A. Recent Advances and Future Research Directions for Hearing Loss Treatment Based on Nanoparticles. *J. Nanomater.* **2022**, *2022*, 7794384. [CrossRef]

11. Mittal, R.; Pena, S.A.; Zhu, A.; Eshraghi, N.; Fesharaki, A.; Horesh, E.J.; Mittal, J.; Eshraghi, A.A. Nanoparticle-Based Drug Delivery in the Inner Ear: Current Challenges, Limitations and Opportunities. *Artif. Cells Nanomed. Biotechnol.* **2019**, *47*, 1312–1320. [CrossRef] [PubMed]
12. Lin, Y.C.; Shih, C.P.; Chen, H.C.; Chou, Y.L.; Sytwu, H.K.; Fang, M.C.; Lin, Y.Y.; Kuo, C.Y.; Su, H.H.; Hung, C.L.; et al. Ultrasound Microbubble–Facilitated Inner Ear Delivery of Gold Nanoparticles Involves Transient Disruption of the Tight Junction Barrier in the Round Window Membrane. *Front. Pharmacol.* **2021**, *12*, 689546. [CrossRef] [PubMed]
13. Mahdi, W.A.; Hussain, A.; Ramzan, M.; Faruk, A.; Bukhari, S.I.; Dev, A. Pluronic-Coated Biogenic Gold Nanoparticles for Colon Delivery of 5-Fluorouracil: In Vitro and Ex Vivo Studies. *AAPS PharmSciTech* **2021**, *22*, 64. [CrossRef] [PubMed]
14. Fenwick, N.; Griffin, G.; Gauthier, C. The Welfare of Animals Used in Science: How the "Three Rs" Ethic Guides Improvements. *Can. Vet. J.* **2009**, *50*, 523–530. [PubMed]
15. Frens, G. Controlled Nucleation for the Regulation of the Particle Size in Monodisperse Gold Suspensions. *Nat. Phys. Sci.* **1973**, *241*, 20–22. [CrossRef]
16. Ruebhausen, M.R.; Brozoski, T.J.; Bauer, C.A. A Comparison of the Effects of Isoflurane and Ketamine Anesthesia on Auditory Brainstem Response (ABR) Thresholds in Rats. *Hear. Res.* **2012**, *287*, 25–29. [CrossRef]
17. Tamames, I.; King, C.; Bas, E.; Dietrich, W.D.; Telischi, F.; Rajguru, S.M. A Cool Approach to Reducing Electrode-Induced Trauma: Localized Therapeutic Hypothermia Conserves Residual Hearing in Cochlear Implantation. *Hear. Res.* **2016**, *339*, 32–39. [CrossRef]
18. Gur, H.; Alimoglu, Y.; Duzenli, U.; Korkmaz, S.; Inan, S.; Olgun, L. The Effect of Local Application of Insulin-like Growth Factor for Prevention of Inner-Ear Damage Caused by Electrode Trauma. *J. Laryngol. Otol.* **2017**, *131*, 245–252. [CrossRef]
19. Parys, Q.A.; Van Bulck, P.; Loos, E.; Verhaert, N. Inner Ear Pharmacotherapy for Residual Hearing Preservation in Cochlear Implant Surgery: A Systematic Review. *Biomolecules* **2022**, *12*, 529. [CrossRef]
20. Lee, M.Y.; Kim, Y.C.; Jang, J.; Jung, J.Y.; Choi, H.; Jang, J.H.; Choung, Y.H. Dexamethasone Delivery for Hearing Preservation in Animal Cochlear Implant Model: Continuity, Long-Term Release, and Fast Release Rate. *Acta Oto-Laryngol.* **2020**, *140*, 705–714. [CrossRef] [PubMed]
21. O'Leary, S.J.; Choi, J.; Brady, K.; Matthews, S.; Ozdowska, K.B.; Payne, M.; McLean, T.; Rousset, A.; Lo, J.; Creber, N.; et al. Systemic Methylprednisolone for Hearing Preservation during Cochlear Implant Surgery: A Double Blinded Placebo-Controlled Trial. *Hear. Res.* **2021**, *404*, 108224. [CrossRef] [PubMed]
22. Skarżyńska, M.B.; Skarżyński, P.H.; Król, B.; Kozieł, M.; Osińska, K.; Gos, E.; Skarżyński, H. Preservation of Hearing Following Cochlear Implantation Using Different Steroid Therapy Regimens: A Prospective Clinical Study. *Med. Sci. Monit.* **2018**, *24*, 2437–2445. [CrossRef] [PubMed]
23. Skarzynska, M.B.; Kolodziejak, A.; Gos, E.; Skarzynski, P.H. The Clinical Effects of Steroids Therapy in the Preserving Residual Hearing after Cochlear Implantation with the OTICON Neuro Zti EVO. *J. Clin. Med.* **2021**, *10*, 2868. [CrossRef]
24. Skarzynska, M.B.; Kolodziejak, A.; Gos, E.; Skarzynski, P.H.; Lorens, A.; Walkowiak, A. The Clinical Effect of Steroid Therapy on Preserving Residual Hearing after Cochlear Implantation with the Advanced Bionics HiRes Ultra 3D Cochlear Implant System. *Life* **2022**, *12*, 486. [CrossRef]
25. Dizaj, S.M.; Lotfipour, F.; Barzegar-Jalali, M.; Zarrintan, M.H.; Adibkia, K. Antimicrobial Activity of the Metals and Metal Oxide Nanoparticles. *Mater. Sci. Eng. C* **2014**, *44*, 278–284. [CrossRef] [PubMed]
26. Kayyali, M.; Brake, L.; Ramsey, A.; Wright, A.; O'Malley, B.; Li, D.D. A Novel Nano-Approach for Targeted Inner Ear Imaging. *J. Nanomed. Nanotechnol.* **2017**, *8*, 456. [CrossRef] [PubMed]
27. Eastwood, H.; Pinder, D.; James, D.; Chang, A.; Galloway, S.; Richardson, R.; O'Leary, S. Permanent and Transient Effects of Locally Delivered N-Acetyl Cysteine in a Guinea Pig Model of Cochlear Implantation. *Hear. Res.* **2010**, *259*, 24–30. [CrossRef] [PubMed]

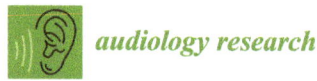

Study Protocol

A Protocol to Investigate Deep Brain Stimulation for Refractory Tinnitus: From Rat Model to the Set-Up of a Human Pilot Study

Gusta van Zwieten [1], Jana V. P. Devos [1,2,3], Sonja A. Kotz [4], Linda Ackermans [1,2], Pia Brinkmann [4], Lobke Dauven [3], Erwin L. J. George [1,3], A. Miranda L. Janssen [5], Bernd Kremer [3], Carsten Leue [6], Michael Schwartze [4], Yasin Temel [1,2], Jasper V. Smit [7] and Marcus L. F. Janssen [1,8,*]

1. School for Mental Health and Neuroscience (MHeNS), Maastricht University, 6229 ER Maastricht, The Netherlands
2. Department of Neurosurgery, Maastricht University Medical Center, 6229 HX Maastricht, The Netherlands
3. Department of Ear Nose and Throat/Head and Neck Surgery, Maastricht University Medical Center, 6229 HX Maastricht, The Netherlands
4. Faculty of Psychology and Neuroscience, Department of Neuropsychology & Psychopharmacology, Maastricht University, 6229 ER Maastricht, The Netherlands
5. Department of Methodology and Statistics, School for Public Health and Primary Care, Maastricht University, 6229 HA Maastricht, The Netherlands
6. Department of Psychiatry and Psychology, Maastricht University Medical Center, 6229 HX Maastricht, The Netherlands
7. Department of Ear Nose and Throat/Head and Neck Surgery, Zuyderland, 6419 PC Heerlen, The Netherlands
8. Department of Clinical Neurophysiology, Maastricht University Medical Center, 6229 HX Maastricht, The Netherlands
* Correspondence: m.janssen@maastrichtuniversity.nl

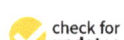

Citation: van Zwieten, G.; Devos, J.V.P.; Kotz, S.A.; Ackermans, L.; Brinkmann, P.; Dauven, L.; George, E.L.J.; Janssen, A.M.L.; Kremer, B.; Leue, C.; et al. A Protocol to Investigate Deep Brain Stimulation for Refractory Tinnitus: From Rat Model to the Set-Up of a Human Pilot Study. *Audiol. Res.* **2023**, *13*, 49–63. https://doi.org/10.3390/audiolres13010005

Academic Editors: Agnieszka Szczepek and Andrea Ciorba

Received: 27 October 2022
Revised: 26 December 2022
Accepted: 27 December 2022
Published: 31 December 2022

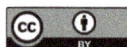

Copyright: © 2022 by the authors. Licensee MDPI, Basel, Switzerland. This article is an open access article distributed under the terms and conditions of the Creative Commons Attribution (CC BY) license (https://creativecommons.org/licenses/by/4.0/).

Abstract: Background: Chronic tinnitus can have an immense impact on quality of life. Despite recent treatment advances, many tinnitus patients remain refractory to them. Preclinical and clinical evidence suggests that deep brain stimulation (DBS) is a promising treatment to suppress tinnitus. In rats, it has been shown in multiple regions of the auditory pathway that DBS can have an alleviating effect on tinnitus. The thalamic medial geniculate body (MGB) takes a key position in the tinnitus network, shows pathophysiological hallmarks of tinnitus, and is readily accessible using stereotaxy. Here, a protocol is described to evaluate the safety and test the therapeutic effects of DBS in the MGB in severe tinnitus sufferers. Methods: Bilateral DBS of the MGB will be applied in a future study in six patients with severe and refractory tinnitus. A double-blinded, randomized 2 × 2 crossover design (stimulation ON and OFF) will be applied, followed by a period of six months of open-label follow-up. The primary focus is to assess safety and feasibility (acceptability). Secondary outcomes assess a potential treatment effect and include tinnitus severity measured by the Tinnitus Functional Index (TFI), tinnitus loudness and distress, hearing, cognitive and psychological functions, quality of life, and neurophysiological characteristics. Discussion: This protocol carefully balances risks and benefits and takes ethical considerations into account. This study will explore the safety and feasibility of DBS in severe refractory tinnitus, through extensive assessment of clinical and neurophysiological outcome measures. Additionally, important insights into the underlying mechanism of tinnitus and hearing function might be revealed. Trial registration: ClinicalTrials.gov NCT03976908 (6 June 2019).

Keywords: deep brain stimulation; tinnitus; MGB; auditory thalamus; randomized controlled trial

1. Introduction

Tinnitus, commonly known as "ringing of the ears", is one of the largest health challenges in the world [1]. According to a recent large survey, approximately 6.4% of Americans experience persistent tinnitus [2]. One in ten patients experiences the most extreme and debilitating form of tinnitus. Sleep deprivation, anxiety, and depression often accompany tinnitus and severely affect the patient's quality of life [3–5]. In turn, this places a huge burden on society, and healthcare costs, and decreases productivity [6].

Subjective tinnitus has a multifactorial origin with heterogeneous patient profiles, which makes it a highly complex condition. The absence of an underlying medical cause in most cases leaves many patients without an available curative evidence-based treatment [7,8]. Tinnitus combined with sensorineural hearing loss might benefit from hearing aids. However, somewhere between 22% and 80% of affected patients are adequately served by using hearing aids [9,10]. The current clinical practice primarily aims at reducing the impact of tinnitus by providing psychoeducation and improving coping strategies via various psychological interventions [11,12].

The etiological and pathophysiological mechanisms of subjective tinnitus are complex and not fully understood. Many investigators feel that in nearly all tinnitus cases, there is some degree of cochlear impairment, leading to diminished auditory nerve activity reaching the cochlear nuclei [13]. Much evidence implicates the head and neck somatosensory system as a separate major factor in the development of tinnitus. It is likely that most tinnitus develops as a result of interactions between these two systems within the central nervous system [14]. According to current theories, tinnitus is associated with increased neural activity in auditory cortices, possibly resulting from maladaptive gating [15,16] and/or an increase in central gain [17]. Specific neural correlates described in tinnitus models are enhanced neuronal synchrony, increased spontaneous firing, and changes in tonotopic organization [18].

A commonly applied neuromodulation technique is deep brain stimulation (DBS). This therapy has been widely used in neurologic and neuropsychiatric disorders such as Parkinson's disease. DBS is generally applied using high-frequency stimulation (>100 Hz), to disrupt pathological neuronal activity and oscillations [19,20]. Hypothetically, this results in an alteration of tinnitus perception and related distress. Further, patients treated with DBS for a movement disorder sometimes also suffered from tinnitus. DBS of non-auditory structures in these patients led to diminished or completely suppressed tinnitus [21–27]. Other implants that could potentially influence tinnitus, and have been investigated, are a cochlear implant (CI) [28] and an auditory brainstem implant (ABI) [29], however, these can only be used in patients with severe hearing loss. In addition, other neuromodulation techniques, such as vagal nerve stimulation [30] and cortical stimulation [31], have been investigated with various degrees of success. These latter treatments can also be used in patients without hearing loss, however, at the moment, there is insufficient evidence to implement these treatments in clinical practice. For a comprehensive review of neuromodulation for tinnitus, see Deklerck et al. [32]. Our hypothesis is that influencing the pathological tinnitus network at any level could be beneficial in theory, but the site at which stimulation is performed strongly influences the outcome. Stimulation in close proximity to the site at which the pathological activity is generated, i.e., within the brainstem [33], might be a more direct and thus efficient target. This could also explain why non-invasive cortical stimulation fails to show conclusive favorable outcomes [34,35].

Preclinically, at multiple levels of the central auditory pathway from cochlear nuclei to the auditory cortex, tinnitus-related neuronal activity is similar to subthalamic nucleus activity in Parkinson's disease, i.e., enhanced spontaneous activity and burst firing [36–39]. The primary role of auditory thalamic neurons is to actively and dynamically shape neural representations of information and to control which information reaches the cerebral cortex [40].

Moreover, preclinical studies support the beneficial effects of DBS on tinnitus when applied in auditory brain areas [21–27]. In Table 1 we listed all currently available animal and human studies that applied DBS for tinnitus. In our lab a rat model for tinnitus was used in order to test DBS as a potential treatment for tinnitus. Noise exposure was used to induce tinnitus in rats after which a gap-prepulse inhibition of the acoustic startle reflex (GPIAS) also known as a gap detection task [41] established the presence of tinnitus. This task exploits the acoustic startle reflex which is present in all mammals and consists of a contraction of the major muscles in response to an unexpected loud noise [42]. A reduction in tinnitus-like behavior was shown when DBS was applied in several structures along the classical auditory pathway, including the dorsal cochlear nucleus [43–45], inferior colliculus [46], and medial geniculate body (MGB) [47]. Importantly, no undesired side effects occurred. DBS of the MGB did not lead to anxiety or disturbed locomotor activity. DBS of the inferior colliculi did not cause any detectable hearing impairment [48]. Other groups also showed beneficial effects in tinnitus behavior in animal rat models, in the caudate [45] and the dorsal cochlear nucleus [44,45]. A similar setup was used as in our studies. These results also indicate that (high-frequency) stimulation anywhere within the pathological tinnitus network could have a beneficial effect on tinnitus [49–51].

Table 1. Overview of preclinical and clinical DBS studies that applied DBS primarily for tinnitus. We only listed studies that primarily treated tinnitus. GPIAS = gap-prepulse inhibition of the acoustic startle reflex; TFI = Tinnitus Functional Index (clinically significant change, i.e., responder = $\geq$ 13 point decrease); THI = Tinnitus Handicap Inventory (clinically significant change, i.e., responder = $\geq$ 20 point decrease).

Reference	Design	Target	N	Uni/Bilateral	Stimulation	Outcome
\multicolumn{7}{c}{Animal (Rodent) Studies}
Van Zwieten et al., 2019 [43]	Noise induced tinnitus, within-subject controlled	Dorsal Cochlear Nucleus	10	Bilateral	Continuous stimulation during test	GPIAS, tinnitus behavior was suppressed
Van Zwieten et al., 2018 [47]	Noise induced tinnitus, within-subject controlled	Medial Geniculate Body	11	Bilateral	Continuous stimulation during test	GPIAS, tinnitus behavior was suppressed
Ahsan et al., 2018 [45]	Noise induced tinnitus, within-subject controlled	Dorsal Cochlear Nucleus	9	Bilateral	Continuous stimulation during test	GPIAS, tinnitus behavior was suppressed
Smit et al., 2016 [46]	Noise induced tinnitus, within-subject controlled	Inferior Colliculus	9	Bilateral	Continuous stimulation during test	GPIAS, tinnitus behavior was suppressed
Luo et al., 2012 [44]	Noise induced tinnitus, within-subject controlled	Dorsal Cochlear Nucleus	6	Unilateral	Continuous stimulation during test	GPIAS, tinnitus behavior was suppressed
Reference	**Design**	**Target**	**N**	**Uni/bilateral**	**Stimulation**	**Outcome**
\multicolumn{7}{c}{Human Studies}
Cheung et al., 2019 [24]	Open-label, nonrandomized trial in refractory tinnitus patients	Caudate Nucleus	6	Bilateral	24 weeks open label	TFI (3 responders), THI (4 responders)
Dijkstra et al., 2018 [25]	Case report in refractory tinnitus patients	Ventral anterior limb of the internal capsule & Nucleus Accumbens	1	Bilateral	1 year	TFI (pre = 74, post = 46), THI (pre = 76, post = 32)

The MGB is a preferred target area as opposed to other auditory subcortical structures [50], as the auditory thalamus is readily accessible in stereotactic surgery. Consequently, targeting the auditory thalamus bears smaller surgical risks and complications such as bleeding and potential neurological deficit. The MGB of the thalamus is a major relay and gateway between the midbrain and cortex, and a core structure in tinnitus pathophysiology [52,53]. Furthermore, the integration of auditory and limbic information occurs within the MGB [54]. Connected limbic structures, such as the amygdala and nucleus accumbens, are related to emotional and attentional symptoms of tinnitus [55]. Hence, the MGB acts as a central hub in networks involved in tinnitus, which makes it a promising structure for neuromodulatory approaches.

Currently, MGB DBS has not been applied in humans. The majority of patients with tinnitus can be treated with non-invasive methods, and only a small number of patients can be considered a candidate for DBS. Based on our pre-clinical findings in rat studies, we developed this protocol for a human pilot study.

The primary objective of the proposed study is to assess the safety and feasibility (acceptability) of bilateral MGB DBS in severe tinnitus. Patients with severe tinnitus who are refractory to the standard treatment program will be included. Secondary outcomes will provide data on the potential efficacy of MGB DBS on tinnitus severity (Tinnitus Functional Index (TFI)), tinnitus loudness, and distress (Visual Analogue Scales (VAS)). Additionally, hearing (audiometry), cognition (neuropsychological test battery), quality of life, and psychological functioning (questionnaires) will be assessed. Furthermore, electrophysiological data will assess fundamental aspects of auditory function and tinnitus pathophysiology. After a successful evaluation of the primary and secondary outcomes in this pilot study, MGB DBS could potentially be further developed as a novel treatment option in severe, refractory tinnitus.

2. Methods

2.1. Study Design

This pilot study uses a double-blind 2 × 2 crossover design in which MGB DBS will be compared to no stimulation (Figure 1).

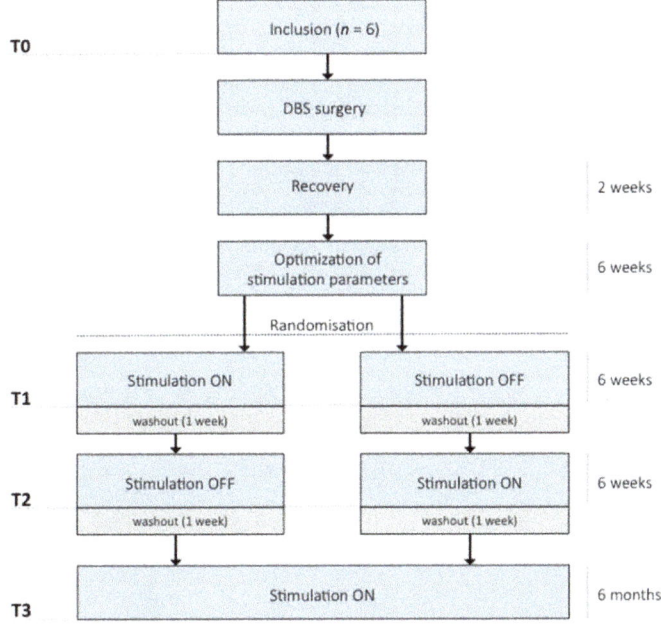

Figure 1. Overview of study design.

2.2. Setting

This study will be carried out at Maastricht University Medical Center (MUMC+) in Maastricht, the Netherlands. MUMC+ is an expertise center for tinnitus, providing integrated multidisciplinary diagnostics and rehabilitation for a wide range of tinnitus patients. The Ear, Nose, and Throat department has long-standing clinical expertise and experience with developing neuromodulative therapies for tinnitus such as intracochlear devices [56]. The neurosurgery department has substantial clinical and preclinical expertise in DBS. In addition to a preclinical DBS research line [57], it is well equipped to conduct clinical trials for new indications of DBS therapy such as Gilles de la Tourette syndrome [58]. Acquisition of neurophysiological data, both intra- and postoperatively is standard practice and is used to unravel neural mechanisms [59].

The study will be conducted according to the principles of the Declaration of Helsinki (Version 10, 2013) and in accordance with the Medical Research Involving Human Subjects Act (in Dutch: 'Wet medisch-wetenschappelijk onderzoek met mensen' (WMO)). This study complied with the CONsolidated Standards Of Reporting Trials (CONSORT) extension statement. Ethics approval was obtained by the institutional review board. Results will be published in an international peer-reviewed scientific journal and presented at scientific meetings.

2.3. Recruitment and Consent

Patients are eligible to enroll if they meet the inclusion and none of the exclusion criteria as outlined in Table 1. All patients will be evaluated and selected by a multidisciplinary team of specialists (otolaryngologists, audiologists, neurosurgeons, neurologists, psychiatrists and psychologists). Diagnostics and treatment are in accordance with national tinnitus guidelines [60]. Based on the Dutch tinnitus guidelines, the tinnitus questionnaire (TQ) is used to determine tinnitus severity [61]. Patients suffer severely (TQ score $\geq$ 47), and are refractory to available treatments including cognitive behavioral therapy and hearing aids in case of hearing loss.

Patients will be recruited at the outpatient clinic of the Ear Nose Throat department. If patients give permission, they receive an information brochure. Two weeks after, researchers will contact the patients to plan a face-to-face meeting. During this meeting, a full understanding of the study protocol is ensured and additional questions are answered. When a patient needs more time to decide, the investigator plans a follow-up appointment after a few weeks. If a patient agrees to participate in the study, informed consent will be signed by the patient and investigator. If the patient meets the criteria, a second outpatient visit will be planned. During this visit, an intake interview will be conducted by one of the researchers, followed by a consultation with both a psychiatrist and a neurosurgeon. Then, the multidisciplinary team will form a collective decision on inclusion or exclusion. Following a positive decision of the multidisciplinary team, a standard clinical workup for DBS surgery will follow. This includes conducting a brain scan and general blood examination. If inclusion criteria are still met, final inclusion will follow. Patients can leave the study at any time for any reason without any consequences. The investigators can decide to withdraw a subject from the study for urgent medical reasons.

2.4. Outcomes

The time frame and methods of data acquisition are displayed in Figure 1 and Table 2, respectively.

2.4.1. Primary Outcomes

The primary focus of this pilot study is to assess safety and feasibility. Safety will be assessed by reporting the rate and grade of all surgical and stimulation induced adverse events in the study sample during the study period. Feasibility will be assessed in terms of the acceptability of the intervention, by taking qualitative interviews at all major time points (T0, T1, T2, T3; see Table 3), and by comparing satisfaction during sham stimulation and DBS.

Table 2. Eligibility criteria. TQ, Tinnitus Questionnaire; DBS, Deep Brain Stimulation; CI, Cochlear Implant; ABI, Auditory Brainstem Implant.

Inclusion Criteria	Exclusion Criteria
• Medically refractory tinnitus * • Age 18–69 years • Experiencing tinnitus that is non-pulsatile and uni- or bilateral • Severe tinnitus (TQ score ≥ 47) • Tinnitus, which is chronic (present ≥ two years) and stable (not intermittent ≥ one year) • Average pure tone thresholds for 1, 2 and 4 kHz <60 dB for each ear • Willingness to participate in the study	• Anatomic cause of tinnitus (e.g., vestibular schwannoma, tumor, middle-ear pathology, temporal mandibular disorder) • DSM-V psychiatric disorders, other than depression or anxiety disorder • Depression or anxiety disorder, manifestation before tinnitus onset • Cognitive impairment or coping problems • Active otologic diseases • Pregnancy or breast-feeding • Active suicidal thoughts or recent attempts • Life expectancy lower than two years • Implantable electronic devices that potentially interfere with DBS (CI, ABI, cortical implant) • General contra-indications for MRI or surgery

* Patient does not respond to available tinnitus treatments (e.g., sound enrichment and cognitive behavioral therapy) and is thoroughly evaluated by the multidisciplinary tinnitus team in MUMC+.

2.4.2. Secondary Outcomes

This pilot study will be used to robustly examine the suitability and appropriateness of the secondary outcome measures (e.g., tinnitus severity, hearing function, depression, anxiety, cognitive function, and quality of life) and make necessary changes in preparation for a full trial. Descriptive statistics and confidence intervals will be reported. The small sample size may hinder a statistically significant outcome. Furthermore, changes in neuronal activity will be assessed by comparing electrophysiological measurements during sham stimulation and DBS.

1. Tinnitus severity will be assessed with the Tinnitus Functional Index (TFI) [62]. The TFI is a validated self-report questionnaire that measures the overall severity of tinnitus and provides coverage of multiple tinnitus severity domains. This questionnaire is the most appropriate responsive measure of treatment-related change. The TFI is translated and validated for Dutch native speakers [63].
2. Tinnitus loudness and burden will be measured by VAS. This will be performed three times daily within a week, which is repeated four times during the study. Furthermore, these VAS scores will be used to assess the effect of stimulation on tinnitus during surgery. VAS ratings for tinnitus loudness and burden are often used in both clinical practice and experimental and descriptive research as a measure of subjective symptoms [64]. Both scales have been shown to correlate with the scores on Tinnitus Questionnaires [65].
3. The hearing function will be assessed with pure tone and speech audiometry. These are clinical standard audiometric tests. Furthermore, subjective hearing will be evaluated using patient feedback.
4. Cognitive functioning will be measured using a validated test battery for standard DBS care. These include the Boston Naming Test, Verbal Fluency, Letter Fluency, 15 Words Test, Trail Making Test part A and B, and the Stroop Color-Word Test.
5. Quality of life and psychological functioning will be assessed by the following psychological questionnaires: 36-Item Short Form Health Survey (SF-36), Beck Depression Inventory II (BDI-II), Beck Anxiety Inventory (BAI), and Hospital Anxiety and Depression Scale (HADS).
6. Neurophysiological measurements: electrophysiological data and auditory brainstem responses will be recorded before and after surgery (T0 and recovery) and at the end of treatment periods I and II (T1 and T2). Furthermore, local field potentials (LFP) will be recorded during surgery and before the implantation of the pulse generator. Details are described under 'Neurophysiological assessments'.

Table 3. Schedule of assessments and procedures. T0 is at inclusion. T1 is at the end of the first 6-week treatment period (stimulation ON or OFF). T2 is at the end of the second 6-week treatment period (stimulation OFF or ON). T3 is at the end of the third treatment period of 6 months stimulation ON. MRI, Magnetic Resonance Imaging; CT, Computer Tomography; TFI, Tinnitus Functional Index; VAS, Visual Analogue Scale; ABR, Auditory Brainstem Responses; EEG, Electroencephalography; LFP, Local Field Potentials.

	Inclusion (T0)	Surgery	Recovery	Optimization	Period I (T1)	Washout	Period II (T2)	Washout	Period III (T3)
Visits and Procedures									
Number of Outpatient visits	2			6	1		1		1
Anesthesiology screening	•								
MRI	•								
CT		•							
Outcome Measures									
Tinnitus severity TFI	•			•	•		•		•
Tinnitus loudness and burden: VAS*	•			•	•		•		•
Hearing function: Audiometry	•		•		•		•		•
ABR	•		•		•		•		•
Cognitive functioning **	•				•		•		•
Psychological functioning ***	•				•		•		•
Neurophysiology: EEG	•		•		•				•
LFP		•	•						

* Last week of the period, 3 random times per day. ** Cognitive functioning tests include Boston Naming Test, Verbal and letter fluency, 15 Word Test, Trail Making Test and Stroop Color-Word Test. *** Psychological functioning is assessed using 36-Item Short Form Health Survey (SF-36), Beck Depression Inventory II (BDI-II), Beck Anxiety Inventory (BAI), and Hospital Anxiety and Depression Scale (HADS).

Dependent on the results of the primary and secondary outcomes, future implementation procedures might be adapted or in case of adverse events, terminated. These adaptations depend not only on the feedback of the individual participants but also on expert judgment. For example, in case the patients describe the questionnaire procedures to be too burdensome, it could be considered to shorten these. Another example, based on expert judgment, could be rethinking the two times six weeks crossover design in case no short-term effects are reported.

3. Intervention

3.1. Implantation of DBS Electrodes and Internal Pulse Generator

A two-staged surgery will be performed. First, bilateral DBS electrodes will be implanted. Tinnitus is a complex disorder for which to date the underlying mechanisms are not entirely clear. The auditory system is organized bilaterally, with a large number of interconnections and information crossing partially (80%) after the cochlear nucleus. To investigate the safety and feasibility bilateral implantation was opted for. Following a standard stereotactic surgical procedure, DBS electrodes will be inserted in the MGB of the thalamus and monitored by radiological and electrophysiological measures. The placement will be conducted under local anesthesia. A CT cerebrum will be carried out and fused with a pre-operative MRI in order to plan the exact trajectory. First, a micro-electrode (InoMed, Emmendingen, Germany) will be inserted. Neurophysiological recordings will be performed in 0.5 to 1 mm steps from 10 mm above and maximally 5 mm below the target with a multi-channel system (InoMed, Emmendingen, Germany) [66]. Simultaneously, at each step, a sequence of auditory stimuli will be presented, which is designed based on known signal processing characteristics of the thalamus [67] and to maximize the likelihood of evoking a reliable response. The amplitude of these responses relative to the spontaneous activity will be used to confirm electrode placement. After the identification of the ventral and dorsal border of the MGB, test stimulation will be applied using 130 Hz, a pulse width of 120 µs and a voltage starting from 0.5 V up to 5 V, or until undesired side effects occur. Stimulation is monopolar, the deepest contact of the electrode is the anode and the battery is the cathode. Stimulation amplitude will be adjusted stepwise. The patient will be asked repeatedly to rate the loudness and burden of the tinnitus sound using VAS. Furthermore, the neurologist will test for undesired side effects. The stimulation electrode will be placed once an optimal effect and acceptable or absent side effects are reached. After placement and fixation of both stimulation electrodes (Medtronic, model 3389) the stereotactic frame will be removed and electrodes will be externalized to enable the recording of LFPs postoperatively.

After surgery, the patient will be transferred to a neurosurgical medium care unit. On the second post-operative day a CT cerebrum will be made to confirm the definite electrode positioning. After one or two days the pulse generator (Medtronic, Activa PC model 37601) will be subcutaneously placed under general anesthesia and the electrodes will be connected. One or two days postoperative, the patient can be discharged. After the end of the trial, follow-up as standard DBS care will be provided.

3.2. Stimulation Parameters

Based on the results in rats it is expected that only high-frequency stimulation will be effective for tinnitus reduction [43]. The following stimulation parameters will be used as the minimum and maximum values during the optimization period to determine optimal stimulation parameters: stimulation frequency (2–200 Hz), pulse width (60–450 µs), and voltage (starting from 0 to a maximum of 5 V). Initially, the stimulation will be bilateral with the same parameters on both sides. Voltages will be increased symmetrically depending on the clinical effect and side effects. In case of stimulation induced side effects, bilateral stimulation can be adapted to unilateral stimulation. During treatment, patients will visit the outpatient clinic weekly. During this period, side effects and tolerability of the stimulation in daily life are evaluated; however, no instant change in tinnitus is expected due to the complexity of the disorder and the anticipated burden and duration of tinnitus. Following the treatment episode, there will be a one-week period for washout of a possible residual therapeutic effect.

3.3. Neurophysiological Assessments

EEG will be recorded with surface electrodes applied to the scalp in accordance with the 10–20 international system standard. Just before the implantation of the pulse generator, cables are externalized, which enables simultaneous recordings of LFPs from the depth electrodes in the MGB.

For each session, several recordings with and without auditory stimulation will be obtained. In the first phase, resting-state activity will be recorded with eyes open and eyes closed. These initial recordings serve to establish baselines for task-independent neural oscillatory activity, network activity, and coherence (assessed on the basis of dominant spontaneous low-frequency oscillations and their variability). In the second phase, auditory brainstem responses will be recorded using a standard protocol to probe auditory brainstem function before and after surgery. In the third phase, activity will be recorded during experimental auditory stimulation. The respective measures will allow assessing of basic characteristics of auditory function in general, and sensory gating in particular (i.e., adaptive filtering based on predictable feature-based and temporal information) in accordance with the adopted model. These measures have been previously obtained via surface EEG recordings in humans [68,69] and preliminary data show comparable responses recorded from the thalamus in the animal model.

Taken together, these measures allow for assessing fundamental signal coding (linear vs. event-related), time-course (temporal relation of thalamic and surface responses), and functional (deviance processing, regularity, predictability, gating) aspects of auditory function. Dysfunctional processing would correspondingly be indexed by desynchronization, lack of suppression effects, temporal decoupling (reduced correlation between thalamic and surface responses), and overall high variability.

3.4. Randomization and Blinding

Randomization will be performed directly after the period of stimulation optimization by an independent institution, the Clinical Trial Center Maastricht (CTCM). Patients will be randomly assigned to one of the two study groups. The investigator who adjusts DBS parameters cannot be blinded. All other investigators and the patient are blinded to the study group. In case the patients are considered unblinded due to the nature of the stimulation the protocol will be carried out as planned. Only in the case of medical concerns, the patient and investigators will be unblinded in order to provide the care needed.

3.5. Data Collection and Management

Data handling will be organized according to the "FAIR guiding principles for scientific data management and stewardship" [70]. This will be carried out in cooperation with the CTCM, which is a local center that facilitates human research. Data will be collected by data entry in Castor electronic data capture (EDC); a cloud-based, password-protected data management system providing a backup on a secured server. Audit trailing provides basic data to backtrack a file to its origin. Paper versions of questionnaires will be kept in a locked closet in the research office. All data will be anonymously coded. The key will be available to the project leader only. Data collection is monitored by the CTCM; a specific monitor is appointed to the study who will follow up on the progress and adherence to the protocol. The monitor will perform periodic checks. A data safety monitoring board, comprising a statistician and two neurologists, is instituted which periodically reviews and evaluates the accumulated study data concerning participant safety, study conduct, progress, and efficacy. The data safety monitoring board receives and reviews the progress and acquired data of this trial and provides the research team with advice on the conduct of the trial.

3.6. Statistical Analyses

The safety and feasibility outcomes will be reported descriptively. Descriptive statistics with 95% confidence intervals will be used to present preliminary data of secondary outcomes such as tinnitus (severity, loudness and distress), anxiety, depression, hearing function, quality of life, and cognitive functioning. These data will provide some insight into population characteristics and might indicate potential changes in mean scores between the intervention and sham stimulation.

3.7. Sample Size

As this is a pilot study, no formal sample size calculation was performed. Only a small sample size will be used because a large burden is being placed on the participants. Additionally, there is uncertainty about potential benefits and the fact that the effects of surgery are still unknown, even though it is expected to be safe. Based on previous first-in-human DBS studies [24,58,71], we expect to adequately address the safety and the proof of concept purpose of the study by including six patients. In these invasive first-in-human trial small sample sizes are not uncommon. Furthermore, this number of patients will enable the collection of preliminary results that will provide meaningful information about the differences between the intervention and sham stimulation. In case of the withdrawal of a patient or in case of incomplete data there will be no replacement of individual participants.

3.8. Patient and Public Involvement

Patients from the Dutch tinnitus support group were involved in the development of this protocol. During information meetings, aspects of the study were discussed such as feasibility and eligibility criteria. Furthermore, patients were involved in the development of patient information.

4. Discussion

One of the main ethical considerations in this study is balancing risks and benefits. The potential benefit of the intervention is a reduction of tinnitus loudness and tinnitus burden. Risks of this minimally invasive and reversible form of functional neurosurgery are surgery-related complications (e.g., cerebral hemorrhage or infarction, CSF leak, seizures, meningitis or encephalitis), hardware failure (e.g., lead rupture, extension fibrosis, device migration) and stimulation related side effects. These latter effects are unknown as clinical MGB DBS has not been performed before. The function of the MGB is primarily hearing thus other side effects than hearing-related effects are less likely. Animal studies did not show hearing loss, anxiety or locomotion-related side effects in DBS in subcortical auditory structures [43,47,48]. We also reviewed possible side effects based on the brain structures surrounding the MGB. The MGB is located posterior to the subthalamic nucleus. The MGB is 8mm wide, 6mm long and 6.5mm high with its largest volume at -3.5mm from the AC-PC (anterior commissure-posterior commissure) plane. Considering the relatively large size of the MGB, current spread outside the MGB is unlikely if the DBS electrode is positioned in the center. Neighboring structures of the MGB are structures similar to other commonly used stimulation targets. The current spread to the anterior side of the MGB could result in internal capsule effects. These side effects are known from subthalamic nucleus (STN) DBS treatment for dystonia and Parkinson's disease. The possible side effects of internal capsule stimulation are dysarthria, muscle contractions, and gaze paresis. Posterior to the MGB the ventricle can be found. Possible side effects are known from anterior nucleus of the thalamus (ANT) DBS which has also a border at the ventricle. Antero-medially the sensory thalamus is located which is targeted when performing DBS to treat pain. More medially the fields of Forel are located. Possible side effects are known from STN DBS in which current spread also may occur to the fields of Forel which can result in disturbances of speech, postural stability and gait. Laterally to the MGB the optic tract is located. We know from globus pallidus internus (GPi) DBS that stimulation of the optic tract elicits phosphenes. All these side effects from current spread to surrounding regions are elicited by stimulation and thus reversible. Taking this together, MGB DBS could induce changes in auditory sensation, and there is a slight risk for side effects due to current spread. In case of undesired side effects, stimulation parameters can be adapted or stimulation can be turned off. The principal investigator will immediately inform the data safety monitoring board and the medical ethical committee in case of serious side effect.

In relation to correctly and carefully evaluating risks and benefits, patient recruitment and extensive informed consent are crucial steps. The primary inclusion criterion is that patients need to be refractory to current treatment (e.g., cognitive behavioral therapy); second, sufficient hearing is required and patients cannot be candidates for cochlear implants. In a refractory patient population, patient selection is an important factor. Patients should have gone through all available proven treatments without significant success. This treatment could be the last resort for these patients when all else has failed. However, this could also affect their decision-making, making them eager to participate in the hopes of a cure. Therefore, patients should be informed about the implications and the uncertainties concerning the outcome extensively during the informed consent procedure. Thus, creating realistic outcome expectations and emphasizing the potential effects or the potential absence thereof. To evaluate whether a patient will be able to cope with a potential negative outcome (no result or side effects) a multidisciplinary team is involved in this study. Additionally, both the potential health benefits as well as the scientific gain need to outweigh the possible risks. In order to maximize the scientific benefit one should try to gather as much information as possible to expand the fundamental knowledge. The potential health benefit should be aimed at increasing the participant's quality of life. For this reason, a balance needs to be struck to obtain the most beneficial situation for both science and the participant [72].

A questionnaire study showed that about 20% of general tinnitus patients are willing to undergo DBS surgery in case of a 50% chance of successful treatment. The willingness increased with the number of therapies already tried [73]. Further, patients would be willing to pay 20 times their monthly income to be treated. Most patients would accept a risk of mild side effects, and almost half of the patients would accept a risk of severe side effects [73]. A caveat in patient selection is that desperate patients might see this experimental treatment as a last resort and rush through the informed consent [74]. These circumstances make this group of patients vulnerable and inclusion should carefully be contemplated when informed consent is discussed. Included patients will receive a heavy burden by undergoing a surgical treatment that could be perceived as a last remedy. This could potentially lead to a bias based on effort justification. We aim to minimize the bias by using a combined crossover and randomized double-blind design. The crossover ensures that every patient receives each treatment in a different order, counterbalancing the treatment phases. The double-blind randomization ensures that neither the participant nor the researcher can influence the outcome as they are unaware of the condition. The rationale of the study is for the majority based on animal studies. The assessment of tinnitus in rats (GPIAS) and the method for DBS is at least not fully translatable to humans. An additional limitation is that generalizability to the target group of severely affected tinnitus patients might be challenging due to the heterogeneous nature of tinnitus and the small sample size of this pilot feasibility trial. Still, by carefully evaluating safety and feasibility in this pilot study, we will be able to determine how MGB DBS is received by participants, and optimize a follow-up study in terms of patient support, patient inclusion, surgical procedure and choice of stimulation parameters.

5. Trial Status

Recruitment starts in 2020 and last follow-up is estimated to be completed in 2023.

Author Contributions: All authors contributed to the overall study design and specific methodologies. J.V.S. and M.L.F.J. are leading the trial coordination and helped to conceive the project. G.v.Z., J.V.P.D., J.V.S. and M.L.F.J. produced the detailed protocol, with input from L.A., P.B., L.D., E.L.J.G., A.M.L.J., B.K., C.L., and Y.T., M.L.F.J., S.A.K. and M.S. designed the neurophysiological assessment of the study. G.v.Z. and J.V.P.D. drafted the manuscript with assistance from S.A.K., J.V.S. and M.L.F.J. All authors have critically read, contributed with inputs and revisions, and approved the final manuscript. All authors have read and agreed to the published version of the manuscript.

Funding: The MUMC+ is the sponsor of the study. The investigators are responsible for study design; collection, management, analysis, and interpretation of data; writing of the report; and the decision to submit the report for publication. No funding from any commercial party is obtained to conduct this study.

Institutional Review Board Statement: Ethics approval was obtained by the institutional review board METC azM/UM (reference number NL67027.068.18 / METC 18-063 version 0.4 dated 06-08-2019). Written, informed consent to participate will be obtained from all participants. Results will be published in a peer-reviewed scientific journal and presented at scientific meetings.

Informed Consent Statement: Not applicable.

Data Availability Statement: Data can only be viewed by the investigators, IGJ and monitors.

Conflicts of Interest: The authors declare no conflict of interest.

List of Abbreviations

DBS	Deep brain stimulation
MGB	Medial geniculate body
TFI	Tinnitus Functional Index
VAS	Visual Analogue Scales
MUMC+	Maastricht University Medical Center
TQ	Tinnitus questionnaire
SF-36	36-Item Short Form Health Survey
BDI-II	Beck Depression Inventory II
BAI	Beck Anxiety Inventory
HADS	Hospital Anxiety and Depression Scale
LFP	Local field potentials
CTCM	Clinical Trial Center Maastricht
EDC	Electronic Data Capture
STN	subthalamic nucleus
AC-PC	Anterior Commissure-Posterior Commissure
ANT	Anterior Nucleus of the Thalamus
GPi	Globus Pallidus Internus

References

1. Henry, J.A.; Dennis, K.C.; Schechter, M.A. General review of tinnitus: Prevalence, mechanisms, effects, and management. *J Speech Lang. Hear. Res.* **2005**, *48*, 1204–1235. [CrossRef]
2. American National Health and Nutrition Examination Survey, Audiometry section (AUQ_G). *Data Documentation, Codebook, and Frequencies.* 2011–2012. Available online: https://wwwn.cdc.gov/Nchs/Nhanes/2011-2012/AUQ_G.htm (accessed on 1 December 2022).
3. Andersson, G.; Freijd, A.; Baguley, D.M.; Idrizbegovic, E. Tinnitus distress, anxiety, depression, and hearing problems among cochlear implant patients with tinnitus. *J. Am. Acad. Audiol.* **2009**, *20*, 315–319. [CrossRef]
4. Langguth, B.; Landgrebe, M.; Kleinjung, T.; Sand, G.P.; Hajak, G. Tinnitus and depression. *World J. Biol. Psychiatry* **2011**, *12*, 489–500. [CrossRef] [PubMed]
5. Zoger, S.; Svedlund, J.; Holgers, K.M. Relationship between tinnitus severity and psychiatric disorders. *Psychosomatics* **2006**, *47*, 282–288. [CrossRef]
6. Maes, I.H.; Cima, R.F.; Vlaeyen, J.W.; Anteunis, L.J.; Joore, M.A. Tinnitus: A cost study. *Ear Hear.* **2013**, *34*, 508–514. [CrossRef] [PubMed]
7. Langguth, B.; Kreuzer, P.M.; Kleinjung, T.; De Ridder, D. Tinnitus: Causes and clinical management. *Lancet Neurol.* **2013**, *12*, 920–930. [CrossRef] [PubMed]

8. Cima, R.F.F.; Mazurek, B.; Haider, H.; Kikidis, D.; Lapira, A.; Noreña, A.; Hoare, D.J. A multidisciplinary European guideline for tinnitus: Diagnostics, assessment, and treatment. *HNO* **2019**, *67* (Suppl. 1), 10–42. [CrossRef] [PubMed]
9. Kochkin, S.; Tyler, R. Tinnitus treatment and the effectiveness of hearing aids: Hearing care professional perceptions. *Hear. Rev.* **2008**, *15*, 14–18.
10. Trotter, M.I.; Donaldson, I. Hearing aids and tinnitus therapy: A 25-year experience. *J. Laryngol. Otol.* **2008**, *122*, 1052–1056. [CrossRef]
11. Jastreboff, P.J. Tinnitus retraining therapy. *Br. J. Audiol.* **1999**, *33*, 68–70.
12. Cima, R.F.; Andersson, G.; Schmidt, C.J.; Henry, J.A. Cognitive-behavioral treatments for tinnitus: A review of the literature. *J. Am. Acad. Audiol.* **2014**, *25*, 29–61. [CrossRef] [PubMed]
13. Eggermont, J.J.; Roberts, L.E. The neuroscience of tinnitus: Understanding abnormal and normal auditory perception. *Front. Syst. Neurosci.* **2012**, *6*, 53. [CrossRef] [PubMed]
14. Levine, R.A.; Nam, E.C.; Oron, Y.; Melcher, J.R. Evidence for a tinnitus subgroup responsive to somatosensory based treatment modalities. *Prog. Brain Res.* **2007**, *166*, 195–207. [PubMed]
15. Durai, M.; Sanders, M.; Kobayashi, K.; Searchfield, G.D. Auditory streaming and prediction in tinnitus sufferers. *Ear Hear.* **2019**, *40*, 345–357. [CrossRef]
16. Rauschecker, J.P.; May, E.S.; Maudoux, A.; Ploner, M. Frontostriatal gating of tinnitus and chronic pain. *Trends Cogn. Sci.* **2015**, *19*, 567–578. [CrossRef] [PubMed]
17. Norena, A.J. An integrative model of tinnitus based on a central gain controlling neural sensitivity. *Neurosci. Biobehav. Rev.* **2011**, *35*, 1089–1109. [CrossRef]
18. Eggermont, J.J. Pathophysiology of tinnitus. *Prog. Brain Res.* **2007**, *166*, 19–35.
19. Grill, W.M.; Snyder, A.N.; Miocinovic, S. Deep brain stimulation creates an informational lesion of the stimulated nucleus. *Neuroreport* **2004**, *15*, 1137–1140. [CrossRef]
20. Chiken, S.; Nambu, A. Disrupting neuronal transmission: Mechanism of DBS? *Front. Syst. Neurosci.* **2014**, *8*, 33. [CrossRef]
21. Cheung, S.W.; Larson, P.S. Tinnitus modulation by deep brain stimulation in locus of caudate neurons (area LC). *Neuroscience* **2010**, *169*, 1768–1778. [CrossRef]
22. Shi, Y.; Burchiel, K.J.; Anderson, V.C.; Martin, W.H. Deep brain stimulation effects in patients with tinnitus. *Otolaryngol. Head Neck Surg.* **2009**, *141*, 285–287. [CrossRef] [PubMed]
23. Smit, J.V.; Janssen, M.L.; Engelhard, M.; de Bie, R.M.; Schuurman, P.R.; Contarino, M.F.; Mosch, A.; Temel, Y.; Stokroos, R. The impact of deep brain stimulation on tinnitus. *Surg. Neurol. Int.* **2016**, *7* (Suppl. 35), S848–S854. [CrossRef] [PubMed]
24. Cheung, S.W.; Racine, C.A.; Henderson-Sabes, J.; Demopoulos, C.; Molinaro, A.M.; Heath, S.; Nagarajan, S.S.; Bourne, A.L.; Rietcheck, J.E.; Wang, S.S.; et al. Phase I trial of caudate deep brain stimulation for treatment-resistant tinnitus. *J. Neurosurg.* **2019**, *133*, 1–10. [CrossRef] [PubMed]
25. Dijkstra, E.; Figee, M.; Schuurman, P.R.; Denys, D. Effective deep brain stimulation of intractable tinnitus: A case study. *Brain Stimul.* **2018**, *11*, 1205–1207. [CrossRef]
26. De Ridder, D.; Joos, K.; Vanneste, S. Anterior cingulate implants for tinnitus: Report of 2 cases. *J. Neurosurg.* **2016**, *124*, 893–901. [CrossRef]
27. Larson, P.S.; Cheung, S.W. Deep brain stimulation in area LC controllably triggers auditory phantom percepts. *Neurosurgery* **2012**, *70*, 398–405; discussion 6. [CrossRef]
28. Arts, R.A.; George, E.L.; Stokroos, R.J.; Vermeire, K. Review: Cochlear implants as a treatment of tinnitus in single-sided deafness. *Curr. Opin. Otolaryngol. Head Neck Surg.* **2012**, *20*, 398–403. [CrossRef]
29. Roberts, D.S.; Otto, S.; Chen, B.; Peng, K.A.; Schwartz, M.S.; Brackmann, D.E.; House, J.W. Tinnitus suppression after auditory brainstem implantation in patients with neurofibromatosis type-2. *Otol. Neurotol.* **2017**, *38*, 118–122. [CrossRef]
30. Stegeman, I.; Velde, H.M.; Robe, P.; Stokroos, R.J.; Smit, A.L. Tinnitus treatment by vagus nerve stimulation: A systematic review. *PLoS ONE* **2021**, *16*, e0247221. [CrossRef]
31. De Ridder, D.; De Mulder, G.; Verstraeten, E.; Van der Kelen, K.; Sunaert, S.; Smits, M. Primary and secondary auditory cortex stimulation for intractable tinnitus. *ORL J. Otorhinolaryngol. Relat. Spec.* **2006**, *68*, 48–54; discussion 5. [CrossRef]
32. Deklerck, A.N.; Marechal, C.; Perez Fernandez, A.M.; Keppler, H.; Van Roost, D.; Dhooge, I.J.M. Invasive neuromodulation as a treatment for tinnitus: A systematic review. *Neuromodulation* **2020**, *23*, 451–462. [CrossRef] [PubMed]
33. Kandler, K.; Kaltenbach, J.A.; Godfrey, D.A. The cochlear nucleus as a generator of tinnitus-related signals. In *The Oxford Handbook of the Auditory Brainstem*; Oxford University Press: Oxford, UK, 2019; pp. 188–222.
34. Jacquemin, L.; Mertens, G.; Shekhawat, G.S.; Van de Heyning, P.; Vanderveken, O.M.; Topsakal, V. High definition transcranial direct current stimulation (HD-tDCS) for chronic tinnitus: Outcomes from a prospective longitudinal large cohort study. *Prog. Brain Res.* **2021**, *263*, 137–152. [PubMed]
35. Hoekstra, C.E.; Versnel, H.; Neggers, S.F.; Niesten, M.E.; van Zanten, G.A. Bilateral low-frequency repetitive transcranial magnetic stimulation of the auditory cortex in tinnitus patients is not effective: A randomised controlled trial. *Audiol. Neuro Otol.* **2013**, *18*, 362–373. [CrossRef]
36. Bergman, H.; Wichmann, T.; Karmon, B.; DeLong, M.R. The primate subthalamic nucleus. II. Neuronal activity in the MPTP model of parkinsonism. *J. Neurophysiol.* **1994**, *72*, 507–520. [CrossRef] [PubMed]

37. Benazzouz, A.; Breit, S.; Koudsie, A.; Pollak, P.; Krack, P.; Benabid, A.L. Intraoperative microrecordings of the subthalamic nucleus in Parkinson's disease. *Mov. Disord.* **2002**, *17* (Suppl. 3), S145–S149. [CrossRef]
38. Janssen, M.L.; Zwartjes, D.G.; Tan, S.K.; Vlamings, R.; Jahanshahi, A.; Heida, T.; Hoogland, G.; Steinbusch, H.W.; Visser-Vandewalle, V.; Temel, Y. Mild dopaminergic lesions are accompanied by robust changes in subthalamic nucleus activity. *Neurosci. Lett.* **2012**, *508*, 101–105. [CrossRef]
39. Kalappa, B.I.; Brozoski, T.J.; Turner, J.G.; Caspary, D.M. Single unit hyperactivity and bursting in the auditory thalamus of awake rats directly correlates with behavioural evidence of tinnitus. *J. Physiol.* **2014**, *592*, 5065–5078. [CrossRef]
40. Bartlett, E.L. The organization and physiology of the auditory thalamus and its role in processing acoustic features important for speech perception. *Brain Lang.* **2013**, *126*, 29–48. [CrossRef]
41. Turner, J.G.; Brozoski, T.J.; Bauer, C.A.; Parrish, J.L.; Myers, K.; Hughes, L.F.; Caspary, D.M. Gap detection deficits in rats with tinnitus: A potential novel screening tool. *Behav. Neurosci.* **2006**, *120*, 188–195. [CrossRef]
42. Koch, M. The neurobiology of startle. *Prog. Neurobiol.* **1999**, *59*, 107–128. [CrossRef]
43. Van Zwieten, G.; Jahanshahi, A.; van Erp, M.L.; Temel, Y.; Stokroos, R.J.; Janssen, M.L.F. Alleviation of tinnitus with high-frequency stimulation of the dorsal cochlear nucleus: A rodent study. *Trends Hear.* **2019**, *23*, 2331216519835080. [CrossRef]
44. Luo, H.; Zhang, X.; Nation, J.; Pace, E.; Lepczyk, L.; Zhang, J. Tinnitus suppression by electrical stimulation of the rat dorsal cochlear nucleus. *Neurosci. Lett.* **2012**, *522*, 16–20. [CrossRef] [PubMed]
45. Ahsan, S.F.; Luo, H.; Zhang, J.; Kim, E.; Xu, Y. An animal model of deep brain stimulation for treating tinnitus: A proof of concept study. *Laryngoscope* **2018**, *128*, 1213–1222. [CrossRef]
46. Smit, J.V.; Janssen, M.L.; van Zwieten, G.; Jahanshahi, A.; Temel, Y.; Stokroos, R.J. Deep brain stimulation of the inferior colliculus in the rodent suppresses tinnitus. *Brain Res.* **2016**, *1650*, 118–124. [CrossRef] [PubMed]
47. Van Zwieten, G.; Janssen, M.L.F.; Smit, J.V.; Janssen, A.M.L.; Roet, M.; Jahanshahi, A. Inhibition of experimental tinnitus with high frequency stimulation of the rat medial geniculate body. *Neuromodulation* **2018**, *22*, 416–424. [CrossRef]
48. Smit, J.V.; Jahanshahi, A.; Janssen, M.L.F.; Stokroos, R.J.; Temel, Y. Hearing assessment during deep brain stimulation of the central nucleus of the inferior colliculus and dentate cerebellar nucleus in rat. *PeerJ* **2017**, *5*, e3892. [CrossRef] [PubMed]
49. Smit, J.V.; Janssen, M.L.; Schulze, H.; Jahanshahi, A.; Van Overbeeke, J.J.; Temel, Y.; Stokroos, R. Deep brain stimulation in tinnitus: Current and future perspectives. *Brain Res.* **2015**, *1608*, 51–65. [CrossRef] [PubMed]
50. Van Zwieten, G.; Smit, J.V.; Jahanshahi, A.; Temel, Y.; Stokroos, R.J. Tinnitus: Is there a place for brain stimulation? *Surg. Neurol. Int.* **2016**, *7* (Suppl. 4), S125–S129. [CrossRef] [PubMed]
51. Rammo, R.; Ali, R.; Pabaney, A.; Seidman, M.; Schwalb, J. Surgical neuromodulation of tinnitus: A review of current therapies and future applications. *Neuromodulation* **2018**, *22*, 380–387. [CrossRef]
52. Leaver, A.M.; Renier, L.; Chevillet, M.A.; Morgan, S.; Kim, H.J.; Rauschecker, J.P. Dysregulation of limbic and auditory networks in tinnitus. *Neuron* **2011**, *69*, 33–43. [CrossRef]
53. Rauschecker, J.P.; Leaver, A.M.; Muhlau, M. Tuning out the noise: Limbic-auditory interactions in tinnitus. *Neuron* **2010**, *66*, 819–826. [CrossRef] [PubMed]
54. Kraus, K.S.; Canlon, B. Neuronal connectivity and interactions between the auditory and limbic systems. Effects of noise and tinnitus. *Hear. Res.* **2012**, *288*, 34–46. [CrossRef] [PubMed]
55. De Ridder, D.; Vanneste, S.; Weisz, N.; Londero, A.; Schlee, W.; Elgoyhen, A.B. An integrative model of auditory phantom perception: Tinnitus as a unified percept of interacting separable subnetworks. *Neurosci. Biobehav. Rev.* **2014**, *44*, 16–32. [CrossRef] [PubMed]
56. Arts, R.A.; George, E.L.; Griessner, A.; Zierhofer, C.; Stokroos, R.J. Tinnitus suppression by intracochlear electrical stimulation in single-sided deafness: A prospective clinical trial—Part I. *Audiol. Neuro Otol.* **2015**, *20*, 294–313. [CrossRef] [PubMed]
57. Tan, S.; Vlamings, R.; Lim, L.; Sesia, T.; Janssen, M.L.; Steinbusch, H.W.; Visser-Vandewalle, V.; Temel, Y. Experimental deep brain stimulation in animal models. *Neurosurgery* **2010**, *67*, 1073–1079; discussion 80. [CrossRef]
58. Ackermans, L.; Duits, A.; van der Linden, C.; Tijssen, M.; Schruers, K.; Temel, Y.; Kleijer, M.; Nederveen, P.; Bruggeman, R.; Tromp, S. Double-blind clinical trial of thalamic stimulation in patients with Tourette syndrome. *Brain* **2011**, *134*, 832–844. [CrossRef]
59. Janssen, M.L.; Zwartjes, D.G.; Temel, Y.; van Kranen-Mastenbroek, V.; Duits, A.; Bour, L.J.; Veltink, P.H.; Heida, T.; Visser-Vandewalle, V. Subthalamic neuronal responses to cortical stimulation. *Mov. Disord.* **2012**, *27*, 435–438. [CrossRef]
60. Joustra, J.; Buwalda, J.; Cima, R.; Free, R.H.; Hofman, R.; De Kleine, E. Dutch Tinnitus Guideline. Richtlijn Tinnitus. Nederlandse Vereniging voor Keel-Neus-Oorheelkunde en Heelkunde van het Hoofd-Halsgebied 2016. Available online: https://richtlijnendatabase.nl/richtlijn/tinnitus/tinnitus_-_startpagina.html (accessed on 1 December 2022).
61. Hallam, R.S.; Jakes, S.C.; Hinchcliffe, R. Cognitive variables in tinnitus annoyance. *Br. J. Clin. Psychol.* **1988**, *27*, 213–222. [CrossRef]
62. Meikle, M.B.; Henry, J.A.; Griest, S.E.; Stewart, B.J.; Abrams, H.B.; McArdle, R. The tinnitus functional index: Development of a new clinical measure for chronic, intrusive tinnitus. *Ear Hear.* **2012**, *33*, 153–176. [CrossRef]
63. Rabau, S.; Wouters, K.; Van de Heyning, P. Validation and translation of the Dutch tinnitus functional index. *B-ENT* **2014**, *10*, 251–258.
64. Cline, M.E.; Herman, J.; Shaw, E.R.; Morton, R.D. Standardization of the visual analogue scale. *Nurs. Res.* **1992**, *41*, 378–380. [CrossRef] [PubMed]

65. Adamchic, I.; Langguth, B.; Hauptmann, C.; Tass, P.A. Psychometric evaluation of visual analog scale for the assessment of chronic tinnitus. *Am. J.Audiol.* **2012**, *21*, 215–225. [CrossRef]
66. Schaper, F.; Zhao, Y.; Janssen, M.L.F.; Wagner, G.L.; Colon, A.J.; Hilkman, D.M.W.; Gommer, E.; Vlooswijk, M.C.G.; Hoogland, G.; Ackermans, L. Single-cell recordings to target the anterior nucleus of the thalamus in deep brain stimulation for patients with refractory epilepsy. *Int. J. Neural. Syst.* **2018**, *29*, 1850012. [CrossRef] [PubMed]
67. Sherman, S.M. Thalamic relay functions. *Prog. Brain Res.* **2001**, *134*, 51–69.
68. Schwartze, M.; Farrugia, N.; Kotz, S.A. Dissociation of formal and temporal predictability in early auditory evoked potentials. *Neuropsychologia* **2013**, *51*, 320–325. [CrossRef]
69. Schwartze, M.; Tavano, A.; Schroger, E.; Kotz, S.A. Temporal aspects of prediction in audition: Cortical and subcortical neural mechanisms. *Int. J. Psychophysiol.* **2012**, *83*, 200–207. [CrossRef]
70. Wilkinson, M.D.; Dumontier, M.; Aalbersberg, I.J.; Appleton, G.; Axton, M.; Baak, A.; Blomberg, N.; Boiten, J.W.; da Silva Santos, L.B.; Bourne, P.E. The FAIR Guiding Principles for scientific data management and stewardship. *Sci. Data* **2016**, *3*, 160018. [CrossRef] [PubMed]
71. Koek, R.J.; Langevin, J.P.; Krahl, S.E.; Kosoyan, H.J.; Schwartz, H.N.; Chen, J.W.; Melrose, R.; Mandelkern, M.J.; Sultzer, D. Deep brain stimulation of the basolateral amygdala for treatment-refractory combat post-traumatic stress disorder (PTSD): Study protocol for a pilot randomized controlled trial with blinded, staggered onset of stimulation. *Trials* **2014**, *15*, 356. [CrossRef]
72. Devos, J.V.P.; Temel, Y.; Ackermans, L.; Visser-Vandewalle, V.; Onur, O.A.; Schruers, K.; Smit, J.; Janssen, M.L.F. Methodological considerations for setting up deep brain stimulation studies for new indications. *J. Clin. Med.* **2022**, *11*, 696. [CrossRef]
73. Smit, J.V.; Pielkenrood, B.J.; Arts, R.; Janssen, M.L.; Temel, Y.; Stokroos, R.J. Patient acceptance of invasive treatments for tinnitus. *Am. J. Audiol.* **2018**, *27*, 184–196. [CrossRef]
74. Grant, R.A.; Halpern, C.H.; Baltuch, G.H.; O'Reardon, J.P.; Caplan, A. Ethical considerations in deep brain stimulation for psychiatric illness. *J. Clin. Neurosci.* **2014**, *21*, 1–5. [CrossRef] [PubMed]

Disclaimer/Publisher's Note: The statements, opinions and data contained in all publications are solely those of the individual author(s) and contributor(s) and not of MDPI and/or the editor(s). MDPI and/or the editor(s) disclaim responsibility for any injury to people or property resulting from any ideas, methods, instructions or products referred to in the content.

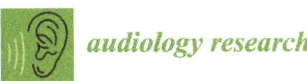

Communication

Tinnitus Education for Audiologists Is a Ship at Sea: Is It Coming or Going?

Marc Fagelson [1,2]

1. Department of Audiology and Speech Language Pathology, East Tennessee State University, Johnson City, TN 37614, USA; fagelson@etsu.edu
2. James H. Quillen Mountain Home VAMC, Johnson City, TN 37684, USA

Abstract: Subjective tinnitus is a highly prevalent sound sensation produced in most cases by persistent neural activity in the auditory pathway of the patient. Audiologists should be confident that they can employ elements of sound therapy and related counseling to support patients in coping. However, patients with bothersome tinnitus may be challenged by mental health complications, and they struggle to find adequate care when tinnitus and psychological distress co-occur. Audiologists in many cases lack the confidence to provide in-depth counseling while mental health providers lack basic understanding of tinnitus, its mechanisms, and the elements of audiologic management that could support patients in coping. At the very least, audiologists should be able to explain the mechanisms involved in and contributing to negative tinnitus effects, conduct valid measures of these effects, and offer reasonable options for managing the consequences linked by the patient to bothersome tinnitus and sound-related sensations. This brief communication summarizes the current state of tinnitus-related opportunities offered in US audiology training programs, and the substantial need to improve both the education of practitioners and the delivery of services to patients in need.

Keywords: tinnitus; cognitive behavioral therapy; self-efficacy; doctor of audiology

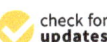

Citation: Fagelson, M. Tinnitus Education for Audiologists Is a Ship at Sea: Is It Coming or Going?. *Audiol. Res.* 2023, *13*, 389–397. https://doi.org/10.3390/audiolres13030034

Academic Editor: Agnieszka Szczepek

Received: 21 April 2023
Revised: 17 May 2023
Accepted: 22 May 2023
Published: 25 May 2023

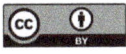

Copyright: © 2023 by the author. Licensee MDPI, Basel, Switzerland. This article is an open access article distributed under the terms and conditions of the Creative Commons Attribution (CC BY) license (https://creativecommons.org/licenses/by/4.0/).

1. Introduction

Subjective tinnitus is not associated with sounds external to the body; however, its onset and detectability may be related to a specific medical condition, such as otosclerosis or otitis media [1], or it can arise from, and provide a reminder of, a specific event such as traumatic acoustic overexposure [2,3]. Tinnitus may also arise as a consequence of ototoxic medication use [4,5]. Subjective tinnitus may appear idiopathically, intermittently, and be unrelated to auditory thresholds [6,7]. Tinnitus often co-occurs with other auditory symptoms such as intolerance to moderate levels of sound (i.e., hyperacusis) or powerful negative emotions such as anger or rage in response to sounds that do not bother other people (i.e., selective sound sensitivity or misophonia) [8]. The diversity of these experiences, triggers, and consequences challenges providers as patients require counseling not only for audiologic rehabilitation, but often interventions for co-occurring mental health complications.

The education of practitioners in this area of audiology is of obvious value, and although published standards [9] reference prevention and management, there remains substantial heterogeneity among audiology programs in the US with regard to classroom and clinical opportunities to study tinnitus and sound tolerance disorders. Reports concluding that psychological management of tinnitus may for many patients provide better outcomes than audiologic management can point both audiology and clinical psychology fields to reasonable interventions (i.e., cognitive behavioral therapy (CBT)) [10]. However, such findings may not encourage audiologists who lack experience and comfort with counseling regarding tinnitus to provide management services for distressed patients. Patients often express frustration and disappointment when seeking clinical services for tinnitus and it is not uncommon for a patient, particularly one who experiences co-occurring mental health disorders, to cease searching despite needing help [11].

2. Methods

This communication summarizes elements of audiology education that can be considered as viable avenues through which programs and students may improve current delivery of tinnitus-related clinical services. Academic and clinical programs routinely assess their resources as they face choices regarding the opportunities they provide. Few programs provide comprehensive and consistent opportunities for their students that meet the needs of patients who have bothersome tinnitus and lack access to dependable care. Current practices in clinical psychology that have relevance and value to audiologists, and that audiologists conduct routinely within their scope of practice, such as fitting hearing aids to reluctant patients and counseling parents of hearing-impaired children, are summarized below.

3. Results

3.1. Tinnitus in the Doctor of Audiology Program

Henry et al. [12] conducted a survey of 75 academic programs offering the AuD degree. The survey focused on class and clinic activity directly supporting tinnitus education and services. In total, 32 out of 75 programs responded to the survey. The results depicted a suboptimal situation in which only a handful of programs (5) specified an hourly total related to tinnitus coursework, while 15/32 programs indicted less than one credit hour (or sixteen total hours of class and clinic time) devoted to tinnitus training. Only 10/32 programs indicated an hourly total commensurate with 1 full-semester course focused on tinnitus, including student clinic assignments that provided contact with patients reporting tinnitus. It may be an overly optimistic interpretation to consider the non-responder programs (i.e., approximately 1/3 of the remaining 43 programs) as offering a similar amount of tinnitus study and opportunities to students.

Henry et al. [12] questioned programs regarding management approaches taught or offered in clinical activity. All but one program indicated instruction/experience related to masking/sound therapy, 91% specified instruction in tinnitus retraining therapy (TRT) [13] and in progressive tinnitus management (PTM) [14]. Other interventions such as tinnitus activities treatment (TAT) [15] and cognitive behavioral therapy (CBT) [16] were specified by programs less often; unfortunately, the Henry et al. [12] summary lacked intervention fidelity information. Therefore, while it was encouraging that at least the responding programs endeavored to support the management of patients with tinnitus, the degree to which their didactic and clinical instruction articulated information essential to the interventions was not assessed. Other interventions specified (pharmacological, counseling, mindfulness, and stress reduction) either required other professionals for implementation, or lacked specific guidelines commensurate with those published for TRT, PTM, CBT, or TAT. Two programs mentioned instruction regarding hearing aid use; however, hearing aid use likely would be implemented as well by those programs specifying masking/sound therapy.

A recent European guideline [10] offered a comprehensive review of diagnostic, assessment, and treatment approaches related to tinnitus patients and providers. The authors identified barriers to and facilitators of tinnitus research and clinical activity, at one point indicating that fewer than 50% of respondents in countries that offered tinnitus services were satisfied with the care they received. Among the barriers, a lack of specialty clinics, a lack of time for counseling and assessment, difficulties related to payment for services, in addition to variability in treatment protocols could be generalized as challenges present concurrently in the US. With regard to facilitators of care, the authors specified among other items the condition's ubiquity, and an awareness that services remain inadequate.

Professional organizations serving audiologists, as well as academic programs and specialty continuing-education outlets, offer additional certification or training opportunities for clinicians. These programs are in most cases offered online, using asynchronous delivery, and employ modules related to different aspects of tinnitus mechanisms and management. Therefore, the challenges of coordinating clinical opportunities with classroom work might not be easily nor reasonably addressed. Ultimately, learners must translate the educational components into routine clinical practice, and while the online programs endeavor to address gaps in training, their effectiveness may be tempered by an unavoidable disconnect if face-to-face clinical opportunities are not provided concurrently.

As the development and delivery of tinnitus programs remains a challenge, their sustainability must also be addressed. The American Speech-Language Hearing Association (ASHA) offered 591 opportunities in the past; however, only three continuing-education "products" [17] are currently available. According to ASHA, it is rare for members to access tinnitus-related opportunities; fewer than ten individuals have completed any tinnitus-related work in the past year. The AudiogyOnline [18] continuing-education service offers 52 options, about half of which are linked directly to manufacturers of devices. Most of the course options on AudiologyOnline indicate reviews of the courses that number from 100 to 2170, hence some courses accommodate thousands of viewers across several years. Most of the courses are indicated as "intermediate"; however, presentation modalities are heterogenous, consisting of videos from academic meetings as well as question and answer text offerings. As with ASHA, continuing education is offered online or as recordings; no opportunities for clinical practice are offered and the numbers of consumers are not easily determined [18]. Salus University offers six 1.5-credit modules that cover tinnitus mechanisms, management, and sound tolerance disorders as part of an Advanced Studies Certificate Program. The modules are optional for students completing Salus' program of study, and are offered entirely online (also offered via AudiologyOnline) and asynchronously in order to maximize availability for international participants.

One notorious barrier to the provision of tinnitus services remains the professionals' remuneration for the clinical endeavor. Fee schedules for tinnitus services provided in clinics whose population contains medicare recipients may reimburse basic, albeit often uninformative measures such as pitch and loudness matching. Many professionals conduct tinnitus-related activity as an ancillary service to, and separate corporate entity from, their routine practice. In such cases, patients are required to pay for services out of pocket, therefore the service will be available to a subset of patients who seek help. Tinnitus and sound tolerance issues, for both patients and providers, highlight many of the US healthcare system's shortcomings; the reimbursement difficulties may represent both a cause and effect of the shortfall of providers and lack of adequate service. It should be noted that, for years, all of the continuing-education and certification training opportunities indicated above were intended to address the shortfall of providers, yet the need remains acute. One additional and widely recognized designator, the Certificate Holder-Tinnitus Management (CH-TM), may support potential providers in a more durable manner and is summarized below.

Considered in the context of Henry et al.'s [12] findings, it is not likely that such basic barriers could be addressed in any reasonable way with fewer than 16 dedicated hours of course and clinic work throughout a multi-year training program offering a doctoral degree.

Perhaps extensive clinic placement opportunities could compensate for the dearth of program credit hours, however Henry et al. [12] reported that only 25/32 responder programs indicated externships that offered tinnitus-related opportunities for practice, or "tinnitus-specific mentorship". Of these, ten indicated that fewer than 25% of the students received such training, while ten indicated that the opportunities were offered to at least half the students; overall, 41% of students received training specific to tinnitus. Tinnitus training outside the University clinic was not consistent, and in nearly half the programs responding, such training was by student request and hence "voluntary". Yet, when the authors asked program administrators, on a 1–10 scale, whether students were well-prepared to offer services, with 10 signifying "exceptionally well-prepared", the responses were for the most part positive with regard to making onward referrals (8.8/10), conducting a tinnitus assessment (7.8/10), providing counseling (6.8/10), and performing at least one tinnitus intervention (5.8/10). If the current regrettable state of tinnitus clinical services in the US is an indication of program efficacy, then there are stark differences between the perceptions of program directors regarding their programs and the willingness with which their graduates approach providing tinnitus-related services. No matter how concerned by our deficiencies we are as providers, it may be that our patients are at the same time substantially more concerned.

3.2. Perspectives on Translation and Interprofessional Practice

If students do not receive a critical mass of experience and information supporting tinnitus management during their matriculation through a program, then it may not be reasonable to expect them to embrace the endeavor in their careers. Indeed, the previous statement has relevance for clinical psychology students, who lack access to tinnitus-related instruction, as well as those in hearing science/audiology programs. Increasing the availability and ability of providers would facilitate the translation of scholarship—particularly clinically directed scholarship—into practice at a rate likely greater than at present. Audiology programs, and their clinical partners, could facilitate this process by employing interprofessional models, such as those employed in group intervention settings [19]. In addition to group options, audiologists could recognize self-efficacy training as an intervention strategy routinely employed in past and current practice with regard to fall prevention, hearing aid use, and audiologic rehabilitation.

The American Board of Audiology introduced in 2018 a certificate program intended to provide practitioners additional training and educational modules associated with clinical practice and the management of tinnitus and sound tolerance disorders [20]. The certificate holder in tinnitus management (CH-TM) completes seven online modules that address the Foundations of Tinnitus Management (tinnitus definitions, management, and business management) and Tinnitus Management Principles in Practice (audiologic evaluation, intervention techniques, and management plans for patients with tinnitus and sound tolerance disorders). Each module requires at least one hour to complete, while some certificate earners use additional time to review notes and study for online evaluations. While the certificate program supports clinical practice in an underserved portion of audiology's scope of practice, and requires completion of module-specific assessments, it cannot ensure that participants have opportunities to practice in a supervised clinical setting. As of this writing, according to Torryn Brazell, the chief operating officer of the American Tinnitus Association (ATA) [21], 483 professionals have earned the CH-TM through the online offering, 435 of whom are audiologists practicing in the US. Approximately 1000 students graduate audiology programs annually; therefore, fewer than 10% of graduates sought the CH-TM since its inception in 2018. The ATA also reported that their AuD degree-holder membership doubled since the certificate was initially offered. It remains unclear whether the increase in certified providers translates into a meaningful increase in services rendered.

At least three graduates from the author's AuD program completed the CH-TM during their first few years post graduation. All three graduates acknowledged the value of having the certificate as a designator affirming their clinical competence; however, the graduates also indicated that the certificate program did not extend in a substantive way the class and clinical experiences provided during their matriculation through the AuD program. As an extension of AuD programs of study, the CH-TM may be considered a welcome addition, but should not be considered a substitute for a rigorous full-semester course supported by a rotation in a tinnitus clinic. If the certificate's completion required two hours/module, then the 14 h total would approximate the typical AuD program time devoted to tinnitus study as reported by Henry et al. [12].

3.3. Audiologists and Non-Audiologic Management Approaches

Other than medical interventions for cases such as otitis media or otosclerosis, tinnitus sensations persist for most patients regardless of attempts to shut the sound off. At present, the strongest evidence base for tinnitus management is CBT [7,10,16], an intervention that convention would state resides outside audiologists' scope of practice. Because there are no reliable cures for the ubiquitous subjective tinnitus sensation experienced by nearly 1 billion humans, research and clinical practice in the area of tinnitus often fail to please providers and patients alike. Because patient education and counseling offer non-invasive tools that may, more than other interventions, improve patient self-efficacy and agency, the need for audiologists to convey relevant, accurate, and helpful information to patients is clear. How best to prepare audiologists to address tinnitus and sound tolerance problems in the clinic, given that psychological interventions have the strongest evidence base, remains a challenge.

The observation that bothersome tinnitus, or "tinnitus disorder" as described by DeRidder et al. [22], would emerge when mental health status is "associated with emotional distress, cognitive dysfunction, and/or autonomic arousal, leading to behavioural changes and functional disability" [22] affirms the putative value of interprofessional care opportunities for affected patients. One barrier to patient care specified by Cima et al. [16] is related to the lack of multidisciplinary teams in some European countries, and a similar lack of opportunities exists in many parts of the US. Without support from other professionals, an audiologist might limit tinnitus clinical activity due to their concern regarding extra-auditory contributors to tinnitus disorder. While such trepidation might seem reasonable, it should be pointed out that audiologists routinely fit hearing aids to anxious and irritated patients who resist the devices. The process is far from high-fidelity CBT; however, it is often effective because it relies upon durable tenets of cognitive training, desensitization, and the establishment of realistic expectations for the patient. Audiologists foster patient self-efficacy when providing counseling regarding fall prevention, assistive devices in classrooms, cochlear implant use, and more. Unfortunately, clinicians do not recognize the similarities between the management strategies they already employ and those that could be of benefit to patients with bothersome tinnitus.

The need for audiology providers to recognize mental health contributions to tinnitus and sound tolerance disorders requires consideration of training components that were viewed in the past as the exclusive purview of clinical psychology training programs. Because tinnitus effects may be exacerbated by co-occurring mental health challenges such as depression or PTSD, audiologists must be prepared to provide onward referrals and appropriate counseling regarding mechanisms shared by tinnitus and mental health status. That tinnitus effects are also compared to those of other conditions such as chronic pain suggests the need to employ patient-centered interventions that support coping and a patient's ability to talk themselves through challenging situations and environments. The evidence supporting cognitive behavioral approaches to tinnitus management [7,10,16] affirms the value of addressing patient beliefs and of supporting patients' understanding of tinnitus to the degree that the patient can employ in a reasonable manner lexical items that support an accurate tinnitus narrative. As specified across decades of studies related to the management of traumatic memories, for example, a patient who can employ accurate and comprehensive narratives will more likely be able to manage the effects of traumatic memories and arousal [2,23–26]. Unfortunately, the lack of preparation offered to audiology students in the majority of AuD programs affects their ability to provide the management strategies and narrative elements required by distressed patients. While it remains unlikely that rank and file audiologists would provide and gain reimbursement for tinnitus-related CBT programs, elements of cognitive training that foster a patient's tinnitus management may be employed. One such strategy, self-efficacy training, sets its focus on improving patients' confidence and agency when confronted with a challenging condition that lacks a simple and accessible cure, such as tinnitus or disorders of sound tolerance.

Self-efficacy training is an intervention with a decades-long history of supporting patients in co-existing with chronic conditions for which management, not curing, is the only option. Bandura [27] offered the rationale and evidence to support specific methods by which patients could be counseled and encouraged to employ thought and action in ways that facilitated overcoming barriers and challenges associated with, for example, healthcare needs or a handicapping health condition. Self-efficacy training [27] supports care by enhancing patients' mastery of challenging activities and experiences, providing vicarious experiences, using verbal persuasion to inform, and improving a patient's sense of control, thereby influencing physiologic and affective states.

Mastery experiences resemble interventions that employ "baby steps" as a way to provide the patient evidence that there are elements of the tinnitus experience that may be controlled. A patient may believe that tinnitus interferes with communication; however, the use of elevated test levels to illustrate the influence of amplification followed by hearing aid evaluation may illustrate that communication can be improved even though a tinnitus sensation remains present. In this case, the patient learns that mastering the use of a hearing aid, Bluetooth streaming device, or other sound generator, although not the same thing as mastering tinnitus, facilitates co-existing with an unwanted tinnitus sensation. Other examples of mastery experiences could include the improvement of sleep through the incremental use of sleep hygiene strategies.

The second self-efficacy objective employs vicarious experiences during which a patient may observe, through other affected individuals, the benefits of counseling, education, device use, or other strategies that reduce distress in others. Group sessions for patients bothered by tinnitus would support this goal as patients would have opportunities to interact with one another, share each other's successes and learn from each other's challenges.

Verbal persuasion is an element of self-efficacy training with which audiologists may feel the most comfortable. Counseling regarding tinnitus mechanisms results from medical assessments that rule out the possibility that tinnitus is a symptom of sinister or terminal illness, and an effective use of communication strategies, for example, may to some degree "persuade" the patient to reassess their prior beliefs and concerns regarding tinnitus and its perceived value.

Finally, self-efficacy training seeks to increase a patient's perception of their own ability to control the influences of tinnitus on daily life, including their emotional reaction to the tinnitus. Interprofessional approaches and teams may facilitate improvements in a patient's coping, and may target elements of tinnitus as it affects emotional and physiologic state. Addressing the patient's sense of control [28], supports a variety of coping strategies that can minimize the intrusiveness and negative effects of tinnitus. In addition to supporting tinnitus management for patients, the inclusion of self-efficacy principles in audiologic rehabilitation classes could provide a reasonable conduit for students to acquire experience and confidence—self-efficacy of their own—with regard to patient care. Note that audiologists taking on the role of a clinical psychologist is not being advocated, and in no way should an audiologist employing mastery experiences, for example, be thought of as conducting a comprehensive self-efficacy training course. The reader is encouraged to consider whether a subset of elements drawn from interventions such as an 8-week CBT program, or a comprehensive self-efficacy training program, provide value to patients in audiology clinics. If the answer is "yes", then it is reasonable to provide students an acknowledgement that clinical psychology employs tools that audiologists (and others) may adapt to improve patient outcomes; at the same time, programs would provide the means and opportunities for students to obtain relevant clinical experience. If the answer is "no", then the practice of audiologic rehabilitation will require recalibration.

A self-efficacy questionnaire intended to assess challenges facing patients with tinnitus was validated [29] and later distinguished the self-efficacy levels across patient groups with and without trauma histories [30]. In those studies, patients with prior military service sought tinnitus-related services at a Veteran's Medical Center (VAMC) audiology clinic. Patients with PTSD diagnoses, and whose tinnitus was related to traumatic exposures—tinnitus with sudden onset that was traced to specific traumatic events—rated their tinnitus handicap and intrusiveness as more severe than patients without PTSD. The questionnaire identified specific elements of a patient's daily routine affected by tinnitus, thereby supporting focused management strategies related to, for example, device use, sleep hygiene, and communication. A student project implementing a guided self-efficacy program intended to improve tinnitus management is currently offered in both individual and group settings at our university tinnitus clinic. Results will emerge over the next few months as the program continues.

3.4. Medical Humanities and Tinnitus Education

Education and clinical practice opportunities related to tinnitus may support the patient's and the clinician's self-efficacy, and the process by which an individual improves their skills may be informed by the tenets of medical humanities. Kirklin [31] described the Medical Humanities program components at the Royal Free and University College Medical School at the University College of London (UCL). The summary emphasized the merging of diverse curricular elements such as the arts, arts therapy, humanities, and philanthropic activities among others, whose addition to student training supported medical management and intervention delivery. Shapiro et al. [32] asserted that the medical humanities have a "moral function" as the practice should compel students and providers to (re)evaluate their attitudes and actions in order to offer patients accurate, thorough, and relatable information that addresses patients' prior knowledge, beliefs, and suffering, as well as their perspectives on healing. The use of the humanities in this context is more applied than it would be as an academic endeavor; when linked to medical practice and service delivery, for example, the arts offer a perspective and a language that may resonate with patients in ways that foster adapting to and managing a challenging condition, perhaps one without a simple cure such as tinnitus. Unfortunately, as pointed out by Shapiro et al. [32] and others, "By and large, medical humanities remain an intriguing sideline in the main project of medical education" [32].

Examples of tinnitus considered in a medical humanities context provide counseling elements that can be employed to great effect with patients. Baguley [33] provided a chapter identifying many instances of tinnitus and disorders of sound tolerance appearing in literature and the arts. Such information may be particularly useful for practitioners who participate in interprofessional teams, who employ self-efficacy elements such as verbal persuasion [27], and who recognize elements related to the medical humanities that may provide unusual and helpful perspectives for a patient struggling with their tinnitus experience. Weaving examples from literature and popular culture into a tinnitus counseling session provides the patient a novel view of tinnitus that may facilitate an understanding of its effects and its ubiquity, not just as a modern-day event, but as a durable element of the human condition.

In a comprehensive book chapter, Stephens placed tinnitus in a historical context [34], and in doing so provided a sort of origin story that can support patient understanding of tinnitus' ubiquity even during periods of human activity that preceded industrialization. By reviewing the Stephens chapter, the provider may address the frustrations of patients who received conflicting or unhelpful information from other clinicians; the chapter affirms that frustrations and fears were shared by patients more than 2000 years ago.

Nothing about acquiring such information cures tinnitus; however, the interaction between patient and provider(s) benefits from the broader scope of counseling topics as well as the likelihood that the expansive view of tinnitus and its effects, when incorporating centuries of art and literature, may become relatable to the patient in a manner that reduces some of the tinnitus distress. If tinnitus existed in society prior to loud sound, if people have been bothered by tinnitus for centuries, and if the tinnitus sensation is so common that it can be used as a trope in movies and literature, then the patient may develop an understanding that the sensation is not unique to them despite the observation that they are the only one who hears it. Medical humanities training and implementation seem an ideal a fit for audiology students and practitioners with regard to supporting a patient's understanding of, and management of, bothersome tinnitus.

4. Conclusions

Barriers to the access and effectiveness of tinnitus interventions continue to challenge patients, students, academic programs, audiologists, and otolaryngologists. It is acknowledged that an inadequate number of AuD programs in the US provide for students a substantive set of experiences focused on tinnitus and disorders of sound tolerance in the classroom and clinic. At the same time, while clinical psychologists employ tools of known benefit to patients with bothersome tinnitus, they cannot be counted upon to address on top of their current caseloads a condition with tinnitus' prevalence. Further, it is more likely that audiologists can gain experience with, and implement on their own, strategies from formal programs such as

CBT and self-efficacy training. The audiologist would employ these techniques much as they already do, as elements of rehabilitation intervention. Greater focus than that offered at present on such management strategies, coupled to comprehensive study of tinnitus mechanisms both audiologic and non-audiologic (i.e., psychological) would if nothing else improve student and clinician self-efficacy. The student who is exposed to patients with bothersome tinnitus, and who collaborates on that patient's management of tinnitus, will be more likely than an unexposed student to work with similar patients in the future. Such opportunities need to be created and fulfilled at a higher rate than at present.

Funding: This research received no external funding.

Institutional Review Board Statement: Not applicable.

Informed Consent Statement: Not applicable.

Data Availability Statement: Not applicable.

Conflicts of Interest: The author declares no conflict of interest.

References

1. Kleinjung, T. Surgical treatment: The ear. In *Textbook of Tinnitus*; Moller, A., Langguth, B., DeRidder, D., Kleinjung, T., Eds.; Springer: New York, NY, USA, 2011; pp. 663–668.
2. Hinton, D.E.; Chhean, D.; Pich, V.; Hofmann, S.G.; Barlow, D.H. Tinnitus among Cambodian refugees: Relationship to PTSD severity. *J. Trauma Stress* **2006**, *19*, 541–546. [CrossRef] [PubMed]
3. Fagelson, M. The association between tinnitus and posttraumatic stress disorder. *Am. J. Audiol.* **2007**, *16*, 107–117. [CrossRef]
4. Eggermont, J.J. On the pathophysiology of tinnitus: A review and a peripheral model. *Hear. Res.* **1990**, *48*, 111–124. [CrossRef] [PubMed]
5. Dille, M.F.; Konrad-Martin, D.; Gallun, F.; Helt, W.J.; Gordon, J.S.; Reavis, K.M.; Bratt, G.W.; Fausti, S.A. Tinnitus onset rates from chemotherapeutic agents and ototoxic antibiotics: Results of a large prospective study. *J. Am. Acad. Audiol.* **2010**, *21*, 409–417. [CrossRef] [PubMed]
6. Baguley, D.; McFerran, D.; Hall, D. Tinnitus. *Lancet* **2013**, *382*, 1600–1607. [CrossRef]
7. Tunkel, D.E.; Bauer, C.A.; Sun, G.H.; Rosenfeld, R.M.; Chandrasekhar, S.S.; Cunningham, E.R., Jr.; Archer, S.M.; Blakley, B.W.; Carter, J.M.; Granieri, E.C.; et al. Clinical practice guideline: Tinnitus. *Otolaryngol.—Head Neck Surg.* **2014**, *151* (Suppl. S2), S1–S40. [CrossRef]
8. Jastreboff, P.J.; Jastreboff, M. Tinnitus retraining therapy (TRT) as a method for treatment of tinnitus and hyperacusis patients. *J. Am. Acad. Audiol.* **2000**, *11*, 156–161. [CrossRef]
9. Council on Academic Accreditation in Audiology and Speech-Language Pathology. Standards for Accreditation of Graduate Education Programs in Audiology and Speech-Language Pathology. 2017. Available online: http://caa.asha.org/wp-content/uploads/Accreditation-Standards-for-Graduate-Programs.pdf (accessed on 5 March 2023).
10. Cima, R.F.F.; Mazurek, B.; Haider, H.; Kikidis, D.; Lapira, A.; Noreña, A.; Hoare, D.J. A multidisciplinary European guideline for tinnitus: Diagnostics, assessment, and treatment. *HNO* **2019**, *67* (Suppl. S1), 10–42. [CrossRef]
11. Bartels, H.; Middel, B.L.; van der Laan, B.F.; Staal, M.J.; Albers, F.W. The Additive Effect of Co-Occurring Anxiety and Depression on Health Status, Quality of Life and Coping Strategies in Help-Seeking Tinnitus Sufferers. *Ear Hear.* **2008**, *29*, 947–956. [CrossRef]
12. Henry, J.A.; Sonstroem, A.; Smith, B.; Grush, L. Survey of Audiology Graduate Programs: Training Students in Tinnitus Management. *Am. J. Audiol.* **2021**, *30*, 22–27. [CrossRef] [PubMed]
13. Jastreboff, P.J. Tinnitus retraining therapy. In *Textbook of Tinnitus*; Moller, A., Langguth, B., DeRidder, D., Kleinjung, T., Eds.; Springer: New York, NY, USA, 2011; pp. 575–596.
14. Henry, J.A.; Thielman, E.J.; Zaugg, T.L.; Kaelin, C.; Schmidt, C.J.; Griest, S.; McMillan, G.P.; Myers, P.; Rivera, I.; Baldwin, R.; et al. Randomized controlled trial in clinical settings to evaluate effectiveness of coping skills education used with Progressive Tinnitus Management. *J. Speech Lang. Hear. Res.* **2017**, *60*, 1378–1397. [CrossRef] [PubMed]
15. Tyler, R.S.; Gogel, S.A.; Gehringer, A.K. Tinnitus activities treatment. *Prog. Brain Res.* **2007**, *166*, 425–434. [CrossRef] [PubMed]
16. Cima, R.F.; Maes, I.H.; Joore, M.A.; Scheyen, D.J.; El Refaie, A.; Baguley, D.M.; Anteunis, L.J.; van Breukelen, G.J.; Vlaeyen, J.W. Specialised treatment based on cognitive behaviour therapy versus usual care for tinnitus: A randomised controlled trial. *Lancet* **2012**, *379*, 1951–1959. [CrossRef]
17. American Speech-Language-Hearing Association Continuing Education Office; (American Speech-Language-Hearing Association Continuing Education Office, Rockville, MD, USA). Personal communication, 2023.
18. AudiologyOnline. Available online: https://www.audiologyonline.com/audiology-ceus/tinnitus-and-hyperacusis/ (accessed on 15 May 2023).
19. Newman, C.W. Sandridge SATinnitus management. In *Adult Audiologic Rehabilitation*; Montano, J.J., Spitzer, J.B., Eds.; Plural Publishing Inc.: San Diego, CA, USA, 2009; pp. 399–444.

20. American Board of Audiology. Handbook: Certificate Holder-Tinnitus Management. Available online: https://www.audiology.org/wp-content/uploads/2021/06/CHTM-HB.draftRV5.pdf (accessed on 12 May 2023).
21. Brazell, T.; (American Tinnitus Association, Washington, DC, USA). Personal communication, 2023.
22. De Ridder, D.; Schlee, W.; Vanneste, S.; Londero, A.; Weisz, N.; Kleinjung, T.; Shekhawat, G.S.; Elgoyhen, A.B.; Song, J.J.; Andersson, G.; et al. Tinnitus and Tinnitus Disorder: Theoretical and Operational Definitions (An international multidisciplinary proposal). *Prog. Brain Res.* **2021**, *260*, 1–25. [CrossRef]
23. Hinton, D.E.; Hinton, S.D.; Reattidara, J.R.; Pich, V.; Pollack, M.H. The 'Multiplex Model' of Somatic Symptoms: Application to Tinnitus among Traumatized Cambodian Refugees. *Transcult. Psychiatry* **2008**, *45*, 287–317. [CrossRef] [PubMed]
24. Shay, J. *Achilles in Vietnam: Combat Trauma and the Undoing of Character*; Scribner: New York, NY, USA, 1994.
25. Herman, J.L. *Trauma and Recovery*; Basic Books: New York, NY, USA, 1997.
26. Brewin, C.R. A cognitive neuroscience account of posttraumatic stress disorder and its treatment. *Behav. Res. Ther.* **2001**, *39*, 373–393. [CrossRef] [PubMed]
27. Bandura, A. *Self-Efficacy: The Exercise of Control*; W. H. Freeman and Company: New York, NY, USA, 1997.
28. Meikle, M.B.; Henry, J.A.; Griest, S.E.; Stewart, B.J.; Abrams, H.B.; McArdle, R.; Myers, P.J.; Newman, C.W.; Sandridge, S.; Turk, D.C.; et al. The Tinnitus Functional Index: Development of a New Clinical Measure for Chronic, Intrusive Tinnitus. *Ear Hear.* **2012**, *33*, 153–176. [CrossRef] [PubMed]
29. Smith, S.L.; Fagelson, M. The Tinnitus Self-Efficacy Questionnaire. *J. Am. Acad. Audiol.* **2011**, *22*, 424–440.
30. Fagelson, M.A.; Smith, S.L. Tinnitus Self-Efficacy and Other Tinnitus Self-Report Variables in Patients with and without Posttraumatic Stress Disorder. *Ear Hear.* **2016**, *37*, 541–546. [CrossRef]
31. Kirklin, D. The Centre for Medical Humanities, Royal Free and University College Medical School, London, England. *Acad. Med.* **2003**, *78*, 1048–1053. [CrossRef]
32. Shapiro, J.; Coulehan, J.; Wear, D.; Montello, M. Medical Humanities and Their Discontents: Definitions, Critiques, and Implications. *Acad. Med.* **2009**, *84*, 192–198. [CrossRef] [PubMed]
33. Baguley, D.M. Tinniitus and hyperacusis in literature, film, and music. In *Tinnitus: Clinical and Research Perspectives*; Baguley, D.M., Fagelson, M., Eds.; Plural Publishing: San Diego, CA, USA, 2016.
34. Stephens, D. A History of Tinnitus. In *Tinnitus Handbook*; Tyler, R., Ed.; Plural Publishing: San Diego, CA, USA, 2000.

Disclaimer/Publisher's Note: The statements, opinions and data contained in all publications are solely those of the individual author(s) and contributor(s) and not of MDPI and/or the editor(s). MDPI and/or the editor(s) disclaim responsibility for any injury to people or property resulting from any ideas, methods, instructions or products referred to in the content.

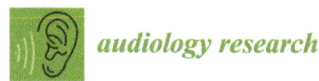

Review

The Ethics of Translational Audiology

Aleksandra Bendowska [1,*,†], Roksana Malak [2,†], Agnieszka Zok [3] and Ewa Baum [1,3]

1. Department of Social Sciences and the Humanities, Poznan University of Medical Sciences, 60-806 Poznan, Poland; ebaum@ump.edu.pl
2. Department and Clinic of Rheumatology, Rehabilitation and Internal Diseases, Poznan University of Medical Sciences, 61-545 Poznan, Poland; rmalak@ump.edu.pl
3. Division of Philosophy of Medicine and Bioethics, Poznan University of Medical Sciences, 60-806 Poznan, Poland; agzok@ump.edu.pl
* Correspondence: abendowska@ump.edu.pl
† These authors contributed equally to this work as the first authors.

Abstract: Translational research moves promising primary research results from the laboratory to practical application. The transition from basic science to clinical research and from clinical research to routine healthcare applications presents many challenges, including ethical. This paper addresses issues in the ethics of translational audiology and discusses the ethical principles that should guide research involving people with hearing loss. Four major ethical principles are defined and explained, which are as follows: beneficence, nonmaleficence, autonomy, and justice. In addition, the authors discuss issues of discrimination and equal access to medical services among people with hearing loss. Despite audiology's broad field of interest, which includes evaluation and treatment of auditory disorders (e.g., deafness, tinnitus, misophonia, or hyperacusis) and balance disorders, this study focuses primarily on deafness and its therapies.

Keywords: ethics; audiology; deafness; translational research

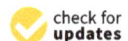

Citation: Bendowska, A.; Malak, R.; Zok, A.; Baum, E. The Ethics of Translational Audiology. *Audiol. Res.* 2022, *12*, 273–280. https://doi.org/10.3390/audiolres12030028

Academic Editor: Agnieszka Szczepek

Received: 30 March 2022
Accepted: 11 May 2022
Published: 13 May 2022

Publisher's Note: MDPI stays neutral with regard to jurisdictional claims in published maps and institutional affiliations.

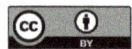

Copyright: © 2022 by the authors. Licensee MDPI, Basel, Switzerland. This article is an open access article distributed under the terms and conditions of the Creative Commons Attribution (CC BY) license (https://creativecommons.org/licenses/by/4.0/).

1. Introduction

Audiology is a large branch of medicine concerned with disorders such as hearing loss, hyperacusis (distorted loudness perception causing several noises unbearable and painfully loud to the affected person [1]), tinnitus (the perception of sounds without actual acoustic stimuli [2]), or misophonia (an emotional reaction to sounds [3]). Another branch of audiology deals with vestibular dysfunctions originating from the inner ear [4–6].

Hearing loss may have congenital or acquired origins [7], and several therapeutic options were developed to treat the affected patients. These options depend on the site of the pathological changes (outer, middle, inner ear; brainstem or central auditory system) and on the degree of the hearing loss (mild, moderate, or severe) [8]. The National Health Service should support people who are hard of hearing and help to early detect hearing impairment [9]. This article focuses on deafness as a disease model and uses that model to discuss the ethical principles in translational audiology.

Translational research is a relatively new but rapidly growing field in biomedical research that aims to transfer scientific discoveries to clinical practice and to analyze clinical observations in the laboratory. Translational research is also referred to as "from bench to bedside". The reverse relationship—"from bedside to table"—is also essential [10]. Many discoveries are made in the clinic by observing a patient's response to treatment. For example, in the clinic, one can observe the correlation of a particular substance, whose biological role we do not understand, with the patient's clinical state. The researchers try to understand its meaning by going back to the laboratory. One can use the knowledge gained to develop a more effective clinical treatment [11]. The core of translational research is synthesizing information obtained from multiple research sources. Such an approach improves our understanding of human physiology, broadens our knowledge of diseases, and accelerates the discovery and testing of new diagnostic and therapeutic methods. The goal of translational research is to increase the quality and efficiency of medical care for patients.

Ethical perspectives recognize that groups of people who are particularly vulnerable to dignity violation and exploitation are marginalized and socially stigmatized, for example, because of illness, substance abuse, poverty, homelessness, ethnicity or cultural identification, or incapacity. However, it is essential to remember that many people who are medically defined as people with disabilities are fully functional. Discrimination can occur due to limiting access to goods or treating people worse by trying to help them against their needs. Considering deafness in this aspect turns out to be extremely important.

Deafness, due to the perceptions and living reality of the person, can be considered in the following two ways: medical and cultural. [12]. In a medical context, deafness refers to hearing loss and, in that context, is written with a lowercase. In a cultural context, to refer to those who primarily communicate through sign language, regardless of hearing ability, often written with a capital letter as Deaf and referred to as "big D" in speech and sign language [13]. Moral dilemmas arising from the multidimensionality of the concept of Deafness seem extremely difficult to resolve; therefore, it is necessary to know both the history of Deafness, related diseases, and existing codes and ethical norms.

2. Deafness in Translational Studies

When conducting translational research with Deaf people, one must also consider the reluctance of this community to participate in genetic testing. This reluctance may stem from the apparent medicalization of deafness, as pointed out by Harlan Lane [14]. This is related to the history of the Deaf, in which genetic engineering methods and medical procedures were used to eliminate deafness. Forced sterilization of Deaf people and conducting genetic testing for congenital deafness are procedures that were used between 1880 and 1950 in the U.S., Britain, and Germany, among others, as elements of the eugenics movement, which aimed to "reduce social burdens" and improve the condition of the human species [15]. To this day, genetic research on deafness in some Deaf communities is met with criticism. In addition, the Deaf community's reluctance and distrust of scientists are compounded by the definition of deafness in biomedical science as a disability, defect and disease. For some deaf communities, deafness might be a unique feature. Despite all the personal and technical aids and the fact that hearing impairment implies functional limitations in social life, the persons are able to organize their social and cultural life, which is why some deaf people do not opt for preventive screenings or treatments to improve their hearing or prevent hearing loss. On the other hand, however, it should also be emphasized that genetic testing can benefit the Deaf community by identifying an increased risk of conditions associated with some types of congenital deafness, such as retinal pigmentary degeneration (e.g., Usher syndrome), facial dysmorphia (e.g., Treacher-Collins syndrome), long QT syndrome (e.g., Jervell andLange-Nielsen syndrome) and renal dysfunction (e.g., Alport syndrome) [16]. Thus, when including a person with deafness in translational research, one should avoid misunderstandings by taking into account the welfare of the research participant. Moreover, the participant's safety should be taken into account by assessing the participant's background, mode of communication, and cultural identification.

This is possible by using the Roman Jakobson's model of the communicative functions of language. Jakobson's diagram includes the following six elements: sender, receiver, message, context, code and contact. The sender sends a message to the receiver. This message has a referential context that the receiver can understand. The context includes all the circumstances accompanying a message that have a key impact on it, e.g., time and place, audience, cultural origin and history. It refers to objects, facts and phenomena from the extra-linguistic world. It is also necessary that the sender and receiver share a common code, by which the first one modifies the message and the second, decodes it. In the case of deaf people, sign language may be a common code with hearing people. The last element is contact, which for Jakobson is a physical channel and a psychological connection between the sender and receiver. This allows to both establish and maintain communication.

In the case of translational research in audiology, we recommend enriching Jakobson's model with ethical principles (Figure 1).

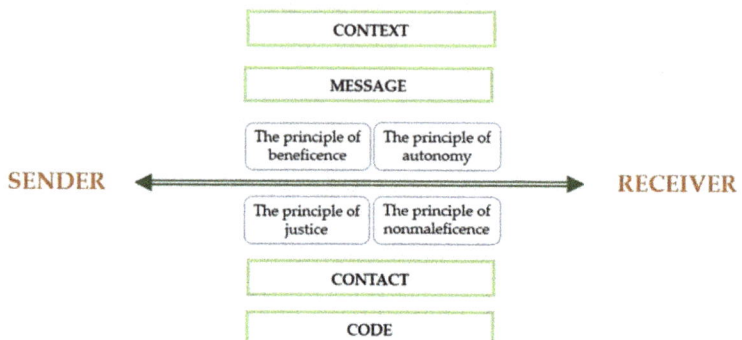

Figure 1. Roman Jakobson's model of the communicative functions of language with ethical principles in translational research in audiology. Source: own elaboration based on Jakobson, R. Linguistics and Poetics. In Style in Language; Sebeok, T., Ed.; M.I.T. Press: Cambridge, USA, 1960; pp. 350–377.

Ethical rules related to the safety of research participants, minimizing harm and abuse of subjects, appeared only in the early 20th century. In 1931, the German Reich published the first ever national set of rules defining the principles for implementing experiments on humans. The document introduced the division of experiments into therapeutic and non-therapeutic. It also emphasized the need to respect the principle of nonmaleficence and beneficence. The regulations included the principle of respecting the autonomy of research participants and obtaining the participant's (or his representative) consent [17]. Unfortunately, this document did not stop Nazi medics from using barbaric experimental methods on concentration camp prisoners.

Nevertheless, the events during World War II contributed to the establishment of bioethics as a science and the development of critical ethical codes. After the Nuremberg Trials, the most significant war criminals were tried, and doctors were directly responsible for unethical experiments. The Nuremberg Code was formulated—10 principles that researchers should follow during experiments on humans. The Code was the first international attempt to define standards of ethics in scientific research and the first document that unambiguously articulated the requirement of obtaining informed consent of the individual to undertake. In addition, in response to the wartime experience, the World Medical Association developed a modern international version of the Hippocratic Oath, the Geneva Declaration [18], and later, in 1964, one of the most critical sets of ethical principles for medical research, the Helsinki Declaration, putting the welfare of research participants first [19]. This principle was not followed during the scandalous observational study of untreated syphilis, the Tuskegee Syphilis Study, which was conducted between 1932 and 1972. The study had racist overtones, as only black, poor, and poorly educated residents of rural Macon County, Alabama, participated. Effective treatment for syphilis was discovered in the early 1950s, yet the study participants were not given treatment, and observation continued [20]. The Tuskegee Syphilis Study disclosure scandal contributed to the United States Congress establishing the National Commission for the Protection of Participants in Biomedical and Behavioral Research. In 1979, this commission published the Belmont Report. This document pointed out the fundamental differences between research activities directed toward the advancement of scientific knowledge and clinical practice focused on the welfare of the individual patient and identified the following three basic principles for the conduct of research involving human participants in medicine: the principle of respect for the person, the principle of beneficence, and the principle of justice.

Over time, these principles have come to be recognized as the fundamental principles of researcher ethics [21].

According to the Belmont Report, respect for the person is expressed in the belief that he or she should be treated as an autonomous agent of action and that persons with diminished autonomy are entitled to protection. Thus, the principle of respect refers to respecting the autonomy of the research participant. Another principle, charity, is understood in the document as an obligation, rather than as an act of kindness or mercy. Two general rules are formulated that provide complementary accounts of acts of kindness thus understood, which are as follows: do no harm, maximize possible benefits, and minimize potential harm. The principle of justice refers to the ethical obligation to treat all people in a manner consistent with what is considered morally proper and speaks to the fair distribution of burdens and benefits that accompany participation to all community members [22].

The four ethical principles, beneficence, nonmaleficence, autonomy, and justice, form the basis for most decision-making in both the research setting and in clinical practice. The following section presents their application both in conducting research in the field of translational audiology and in therapy of people with hearing impairment.

3. Basic Principles of Medical Ethics

3.1. The Principles of Beneficence and Nonmaleficence

The principle of beneficence is the obligation of the physician to act for the benefit of the patient, prevent harm, remove conditions that will cause harm and help persons with disabilities. It is worth emphasizing that, in distinction to nonmaleficence, the language here is one of the positive requirements. The principle calls for not just avoiding harm, but also to benefit patients and to promote their welfare.

The practical application of nonmaleficence is for the physician to analyze the benefits and losses of the proposed interventions and therapies. The physician is obliged by this principle to avoid those that are inappropriate and chose the best procedure for the patient.

The application of the principle of beneficence in clinical trials refers to a researcher's obligation to maximize the benefits of the research and minimize the risk of harm to its participants. Therefore, this principle also includes the principle of nonmaleficence, which sets specific limits for the activities of researchers. It prohibits taking any action that may cause intentional evil or harm to the participants of the research, whereby both physical wrong or harm, i.e., one concerning the state of somatic health, as well as emotional and financial harm, must be included.

A key measure ensuring compliance with the principle of beneficence in scientific research is the analysis and assessment of the risk-benefit ratio of a research participant. Research should not impose risks and burdens disproportionate to the expected benefits of participating in it. In the case of experimental research involving sick persons, which gives participants a chance to obtain a direct diagnostic, therapeutic or prophylactic benefit, the benefit-risk balance of the new intervention cannot be assumed to be less favorable than that of the existing best-proven interventions. In the case of scientific research that does not provide direct diagnostic, therapeutic or prophylactic benefits to participants, the accompanying risk should be estimated proportionally to the scientific value intended to be obtained in connection with the implementation of the study. Such tests are allowed only if they involve risks and burdens that are not greater than acceptable [23].

It should be noted here that participation in scientific research is always associated with the risk of the subject coming to harm. The most frequently mentioned risks include incurring physical, mental, and socioeconomic harm. Research in biomedical sciences often exposes the subject to minor pain, discomfort, or harm caused by medication side effects, and these harms are examples of the physical type of harm. Among the psychological harms, attention should be paid to undesirable changes in the study participants' thought processes and emotional states, e.g., episodes of depression, confusion or hallucinations after taking the drug, feelings of stress, guilt, and loss of self-esteem. These changes may be temporary, recurrent, or permanent. Potential socioeconomic harms include violations of the right to privacy and intimacy of study participants, job loss, and stigmatization. Moreover, information relating to alcohol or drug abuse, mental illness, illegal activities, and sexual behavior creates areas highly prone to abuse [24].

Applying the principle of beneficence and nonmaleficence, the researcher should assess the significance of the potential benefits and harms and, on this basis, decide on the participation of the subject; bearing in mind the principle according to which a research participant should never be the object of an action or a means to achieve an end. However, as an end in itself, the researcher should assess the moral acceptability of his action.

3.2. The Principle of Autonomy

Compliance with the principle of autonomy is based on respecting the patient's opinion and will. It refers to the freedom of the patient to choose the method of treatment and the need to obtain informed consent from the study participants. Autonomy in bioethics and medicine emphasizes respect for the person and their dignity, including the medic, the patient, and the researcher alike.

On the one hand, hearing loss or deafness require a specialist or researcher, who will provide the patient/study participant with information about the procedure, side effects, risks, benefits, costs necessary to make an autonomous decision; on the other hand, the patient or his or her parents have the opportunity to make decisions based on their beliefs and after consulting specialists or other deaf people. The physician or the researcher in his or her actions is guided by evidence-based medicine and the good of the patient/research participant; nevertheless, he or she is obliged to respect the individual's will, even if it is not in line with his or her point of view. Involving the patient in the decision-making process is a desirable phenomenon that proves that the principle of autonomy is respected [25,26].

Regarding audiology and the needs of young patients for implant provision, preserving the child's autonomy is also an essential aspect of medical practice. To maintain the principle of the child's autonomy, with the literal meaning attributed to it, the intervention decision could be postponed until an older age. However, it should be remembered that for the proper sensorimotor and speech development, it is important to take appropriate action as early as possible [27]. It is also crucial for supporting a child's psychosocial development (Figure 2).

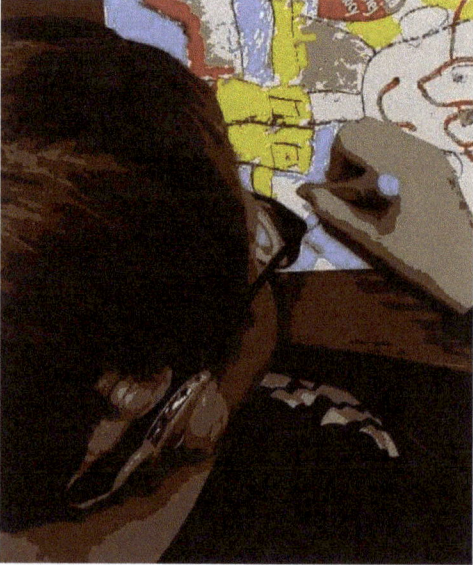

Figure 2. Child with the ear worn cochlear implant processor.

3.3. The Principle of Justice

Another principle of research ethics is the principle of justice. Suppose justice means treating everyone morally and appropriately, including the benefits of participating in the study for all community members. In that case, one should expect equal access for both researchers and, above all, deaf patients to the most modern hearing aids or implants at the best time for a given person. This means that everybody should equally be able to participate in research regardless of, for instance, a gender. Another benefit of participating in research is the application to community members that do not participate in research and to broaden the knowledge and social skills. However, is it so? It seems that both in translational audiology and other fields, especially in modern areas of medicine, the principle of justice functions insufficiently. The application of justice in research should be reflected in social life and the availability of the most appropriate solutions for the patient [28]. Justice in research emphasizes the fundamental principle of "health for all" [27]. This means access to health, regardless of gender, ethnicity, place of birth, political beliefs, religion, economic or social status. Applying the principle of justice in translational audiology could prevent the marginalization of a society. Every researcher in each community would have to provide the best possible equipment implants for the patient, regardless of the patient's place of residence or economic status.

Consequently, each patient would have the same opportunity to develop communication. It does not always have to be verbal communication; this could involve a sign language interpreter. In the context of the principle of justice, it is essential to inform the patient from the very beginning what solutions they are entitled to regarding the implant and what methods of communication they have at their disposal. Researchers in their daily work should apply the principle of justice. A drawback is that this often leads to the study group being less numerous than if patients were only offered one method of assessment and therapy. Therefore, bearing in mind that clinical trials usually have their origin in medical practice, the ideal solution is if the principle of justice accompanies the researcher from the very beginning of their activity, including conceptualization, practice, and research. However, this is not always the case in everyday life. A body that is responsible for safeguarding, so to speak, the principles of ethics, including justice [29], is the bioethics committee. Therefore, an audiologist who is a researcher has several roles in conducting the study. First of all, he or she should take into account the patient's well-being and health, as well as the patient's ethical perspective. Secondly, they must consider factors influencing moral judgment, sensitivity, motivation, courage, and cultural dimensions of ethical practice in audiology [30].

The multifaceted nature of the issues related to deafness also leads to serious moral dilemmas related primarily to reproductive medicine and the treatment of hearing loss. In the case of reproductive medicine, the dilemma may concern the acceptability of donor selection and the selection of an embryo burdened with deafness. Such a situation took place in the USA, where a deaf lesbian couple deliberately created a deaf child. Sharon Duchesneau and Candy McCullough used their sperm donor, a deaf friend with five generations of deafness in his family. Duchesneau and McCullough do not see deafness as a disability. They see being deaf as defining their cultural identity and witness signing as a sophisticated, unique form of communication [31–34]. The moral dilemma concerns the dispute over the understanding of deafness and the concept of care related to the ethical principles discussed above.

Furthermore, although this problem is not new in ethics, a similar situation occurs when parents do not agree to have a child's life saved by refusing blood transfusions because of their faith. For this case also, an extremely current problem of rapidly developing research and gene therapies and their applications should be resolved. The question arises whether genetic testing techniques designed to reduce disease and improve the quality of life can be used to deliberate defective embryos. It should be remembered that deafness does mean not only a lack of hearing, which can actually be perceived in a cultural context, but also several comorbidities, including an increased risk of dementia [35]. This dilemma seems to be difficult to resolve from the principles described above. All perspectives boil down to whether it is good that a sick child has been brought into the world. The arguments from one side point to the use of preimplantation genetic diagnostics as incompatible with its objectives. However, it should be remembered that Gauvin, the son of a pair of deaf women, was born thanks to the knowledge in medical genetics.

4. Conclusions

The idea behind translational research in audiology is to improve the quality of medical care for patients with hearing impairment. Although lofty and deserving of the highest recognition, this idea should never be implemented at an individual's expense in the research procedure. The inalienable dignity of the human being requires researchers and physicians to act for the benefit of the subject, limit the harm, maximize the benefits, and respect the autonomous decisions of the subject. What may serve as signposts indicating the ethical way of conducting translational research in audiology and taking care of patients with hearing impairment are the principles of beneficence, nonmaleficence, autonomy, and justice.

Author Contributions: Conceptualization, A.B., E.B., R.M., and A.Z.; methodology, A.B. and E.B.; writing—original draft preparation, A.B., E.B., A.Z. and R.M.; writing—review and editing, A.B. and R.M.; visualization, A.B. and R.M.; supervision, E.B. All authors have read and agreed to the published version of the manuscript.

Funding: This research received no external funding.

Institutional Review Board Statement: Not applicable.

Informed Consent Statement: Not applicable.

Data Availability Statement: Not applicable.

Conflicts of Interest: The authors declare no conflict of interest.

References

1. Aazh, H.; Knipper, M.; Danesh, A.A.; Cavanna, A.E.; Andersson, L.; Paulin, J.; Schecklmann, M.; Heinonen-Guzejev, M.; Moore, B.C. Insights from the Third International Conference on Hyperacusis: Causes, Evaluation, Diagnosis, and Treatment. *Noise Health* **2018**, *20*, 162–170. [CrossRef]
2. Aazh, H.; Landgrebe, M.; A Danesh, A.; Moore, B.C. Cognitive Behavioral Therapy for Alleviating the Distress Caused By Tinnitus, Hyperacusis And Misophonia: Current Perspectives. *Psychol. Res. Behav. Manag.* **2019**, *12*, 991–1002. [CrossRef]
3. Meltzer, J.B.; Herzfeld, M. Tinnitus, Hyperacusis, and Misophonia Toolbox. *Semin. Hear.* **2014**, *35*, 121–130. [CrossRef]
4. Stach, B.A.; Ramachandran, V. *Clinical Audiology: An Introduction*, 3rd ed.; Plural Publishing: San Diego, CA, USA, 2021; p. 2.
5. O'Reilly, R.C.; Morlet, T.; Cushing, S.L.; Brodsky, J.R. (Eds.) *Manual of Pediatric Balance Disorders*; Plural Publishing: San Diego, CA, USA, 2020.
6. Dougherty, J.M.; Carney, M.; Emmady, P.D. *Vestibular Dysfunction*; StatPearls Publishing: Treasure Island, FL, USA, 2022. Available online: https://www.ncbi.nlm.nih.gov/books/NBK558926/ (accessed on 28 February 2022).
7. Kerr, P.C.; Cowie, R.I.D. Acquired deafness: A multi-dimensional experience. *Br. J. Audiol.* **1997**, *31*, 177–188. [CrossRef]
8. Schilder, A.G.; Chong, L.Y.; Ftouh, S.; Burton, M. Bilateral versus unilateral hearing aids for bilateral hearing impairment in adults. *Cochrane Database Syst. Rev.* **2017**, *2017*, CD012665. [CrossRef]
9. Oliveira, C.; Machado, M.; Zenha, R.; Azevedo, L.; Monteiro, L.; Bicho, A. Surdez Congénita ou Precocemente Adquirida: Do Rastreio ao Seguimento, um Retrato de Portugal. *Acta Med. Port.* **2019**, *32*, 767–775. [CrossRef]
10. Hörig, H.; Pullman, W. From bench to clinic and back: Perspective on the 1st IQPC Translational Research conference. *J. Transl. Med.* **2004**, *2*, 44. [CrossRef]
11. Stelcer, E.; Komarowska, H.; Jopek, K.; Żok, A.; Iżycki, D.; Malińska, A.; Szczepaniak, B.; Komekbai, Z.; Karczewski, M.; Wierzbicki, T.; et al. Biological response of adrenal carcinoma and melanoma cells to mitotane treatment. *Oncol. Lett.* **2022**, *23*, 120. [CrossRef]
12. Levy, N. Deafness, culture, and choice. *J. Med Ethics* **2002**, *28*, 284–285. [CrossRef]
13. Padden, C.; Humphries, T. *Inside Deaf Culture*; Harvard University Press: Cambridge, MA, USA, 2002.
14. Christiansen, J.B.; Lane, H.; Ii, H.L.N. The Mask of Benevolence: Disabling the Deaf Community. *Contemp. Sociol. A J. Rev.* **1993**, *22*, 443. [CrossRef]
15. Lane, H. Ethnicity, ethics, and the deaf-world. *J. Deaf. Stud. Deaf. Educ.* **2005**, *10*, 291–310. [CrossRef] [PubMed]

16. McKee, M.; Schlehofer, D.; Thew, D. Ethical issues in conducting research with deaf populations. *Am. J. Public Health* **2013**, *103*, 2174–2178. [CrossRef] [PubMed]
17. Vollmann, J.; Winau, R. Informed consent in human experimentation before the Nuremberg code. *BMJ* **1996**, *313*, 1445–1447. [CrossRef] [PubMed]
18. World Medical Association, Declaration of Geneva. Available online: https://www.wma.net/policies-post/wma-declaration-of-geneva/ (accessed on 16 February 2022).
19. WMA—The World Medical Association-WMA Declaration of Helsinki—Ethical Principles for Medical Research Involving Human Subjects. Available online: https://www.wma.net/policies-post/wma-declaration-of-helsinki-ethical-principles-for-medical-research-involving-human-subjects/ (accessed on 17 November 2021).
20. Brandt, A.M. Racism and Research: The Case of the Tuskegee Syphilis Study. *Häst. Cent. Rep.* **1978**, *8*, 21–29. [CrossRef]
21. Czarkowski, M. Principles of conducting research involving human participants. In *Bioethics*; Różyńska, J., Chańska, W., Eds.; Wolters Kluwer SA: Warsaw, Poland, 2013; pp. 438–452. (In Polish)
22. The Belmont Report. Ethical Principles and Guidelines for the Protection of Human Subjects of Research. Available online: https://www.hhs.gov/ohrp/regulations-and-policy/belmont-report/index.html (accessed on 16 February 2022).
23. Council for International Organizations of Medical Sciences (CIOMS). *International Ethical Guidelines for Health-Related Research Involving Humans*, 4th ed.; CIOMS: Geneva, Switzerland, 2016; p. 9.
24. National Research Council; Committee on Population. *Proposed Revisions to the Common Rule for the Protection of Human Subjects in the Behavioral and Social Sciences*; National Academies Press: Washington, DC, USA, 2014; p. 59.
25. Salzburg Global Seminar Salzburg statement on shared decision making. *BMJ* **2011**, *342*, d1745. [CrossRef]
26. Elwyn, G.; Frosch, D.; Thomson, R.; Joseph-Williams, N.; Lloyd, A.; Kinnersley, P.; Cording, E.; Tomson, D.; Dodd, C.; Rollnick, S.; et al. Shared Decision Making: A Model for Clinical Practice. *J. Gen. Intern. Med.* **2012**, *27*, 1361–1367. [CrossRef]
27. Rajendran, V.; Roy, F.G. An overview of motor skill performance and balance in hearing impaired children. *Ital. J. Pediatr.* **2011**, *37*, 35. [CrossRef]
28. Pratt, B.; Wild, V.; Barasa, E.; Kamuya, D.; Gilson, L.; Hendl, T.; Molyneux, S. Justice: A key consideration in health policy and systems research ethics. *BMJ Glob. Health* **2020**, *5*, e001942. [CrossRef]
29. Park, M.K.; Lee, B.D. Institutional Review Boards and Bioethical Issues for Otologists and Audiologists. *Korean J. Audiol.* **2012**, *16*, 43–46. [CrossRef]
30. Naudé, A.M.; Bornman, J. A Systematic Review of Ethics Knowledge in Audiology (1980–2010). *Am. J. Audiol.* **2014**, *23*, 151–157. [CrossRef]
31. Savulescu, J. Deaf lesbians, "designer disability," and the future of medicine. *BMJ* **2002**, *325*, 771–773. [CrossRef] [PubMed]
32. Spriggs, M. Lesbian couple create a child who is deaf like them. *J. Med. Ethic.* **2002**, *28*, 283. [CrossRef] [PubMed]
33. Bauman, H.-D.L. Designing Deaf Babies and the Question of Disability. *J. Deaf Stud. Deaf Educ.* **2005**, *10*, 311–315. [CrossRef] [PubMed]
34. Shaw, D. Deaf by design: Disability and impartiality. *Bioethics* **2008**, *22*, 407–413. [CrossRef] [PubMed]
35. Livingston, G.; Huntley, J.; Sommerlad, A.; Ames, D.; Ballard, C.; Banerjee, S.; Brayne, C.; Burns, A.; Cohen-Mansfield, J.; Cooper, C.; et al. Dementia prevention, intervention, and care: 2020 report of the Lancet Commission. *Lancet* **2020**, *396*, 413–446. [CrossRef]

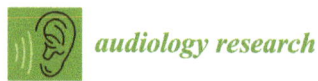

Brief Report

Towards Auditory Profile-Based Hearing-Aid Fittings: BEAR Rationale and Clinical Implementation

Raul Sanchez-Lopez [1,2,3,4,*], Mengfan Wu [2,4,5,6], Michal Fereczkowski [5,6], Sébastien Santurette [7], Monika Baumann [7], Borys Kowalewski [8], Tobias Piechowiak [9], Nikolai Bisgaard [9], Gert Ravn [10], Sreeram Kaithali Narayanan [11], Torsten Dau [1] and Tobias Neher [5,6,*]

1. Hearing Systems Section, Department of Health Technology, Technical University of Denmark, 2800 Kongens Lyngby, Denmark
2. Hearing Sciences, Mental Health and Clinical Neurosciences, School of Medicine, University of Nottingham, Nottingham NG7 2RD, UK
3. Interacoustics Research Unit, 2800 Kongens Lyngby, Denmark
4. National Institute for Health and Care Research (NIHR), Nottingham Biomedical Research Centre, Nottingham NG7 2UH, UK
5. Institute of Clinical Research, Faculty of Health Sciences, University of Southern Denmark, 5230 Odense, Denmark
6. Research Unit for ORL—Head & Neck Surgery and Audiology, Odense University Hospital & University of Southern Denmark, 5230 Odense, Denmark
7. Centre for Applied Audiology Research, Oticon A/S, 2765 Smørum, Denmark
8. WS Audiology A/S, 3540 Lynge, Denmark
9. GN Hearing A/S, 2750 Ballerup, Denmark
10. Force Technology A/S, 2605 Aarhus, Denmark
11. Department of Electronic Systems, Aalborg University, 9220 Aalborg, Denmark

* Correspondence: rsalo@dtu.dk (R.S.-L.); tneher@health.sdu.dk (T.N.)

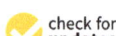

Citation: Sanchez-Lopez, R.; Wu, M.; Fereczkowski, M.; Santurette, S.; Baumann, M.; Kowalewski, B.; Piechowiak, T.; Bisgaard, N.; Ravn, G.; Narayanan, S.K.; et al. Towards Auditory Profile-Based Hearing-Aid Fittings: BEAR Rationale and Clinical Implementation. *Audiol. Res.* 2022, 12, 564–573. https://doi.org/10.3390/audiolres12050055

Academic Editor: Agnieszka Szczepek

Received: 31 August 2022
Accepted: 7 October 2022
Published: 9 October 2022

Publisher's Note: MDPI stays neutral with regard to jurisdictional claims in published maps and institutional affiliations.

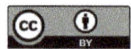

Copyright: © 2022 by the authors. Licensee MDPI, Basel, Switzerland. This article is an open access article distributed under the terms and conditions of the Creative Commons Attribution (CC BY) license (https://creativecommons.org/licenses/by/4.0/).

Abstract: (1) Background: To improve hearing-aid rehabilitation, the Danish 'Better hEAring Rehabilitation' (BEAR) project recently developed methods for individual hearing loss characterization and hearing-aid fitting. Four auditory profiles differing in terms of audiometric hearing loss and suprathreshold hearing abilities were identified. To enable auditory profile-based hearing-aid treatment, a fitting rationale leveraging differences in gain prescription and signal-to-noise (SNR) improvement was developed. This report describes the translation of this rationale to clinical devices supplied by three industrial partners. (2) Methods: Regarding the SNR improvement, advanced feature settings were proposed and verified based on free-field measurements made with an acoustic mannikin fitted with the different hearing aids. Regarding the gain prescription, a clinically feasible fitting tool and procedure based on real-ear gain adjustments were developed. (3) Results: Analyses of the collected real-ear gain and SNR improvement data confirmed the feasibility of the clinical implementation. Differences between the auditory profile-based fitting strategy and a current 'best practice' procedure based on the NAL-NL2 fitting rule were verified and are discussed in terms of limitations and future perspectives. (4) Conclusion: Based on a joint effort from academic and industrial partners, the BEAR fitting rationale was transferred to commercially available hearing aids.

Keywords: audiology; hearing rehabilitation; hearing aid

1. Introduction

Clinical hearing rehabilitation involves the sensory management of a hearing loss, which is typically addressed by means of hearing-aid (HA) fitting based on a set of audiometric thresholds. However, it is well known that there are hearing deficits that are only partially captured by an audiogram [1,2]. As such, conventional amplification cannot be expected to provide effective hearing loss compensation for speech understanding [3,4].

To address this shortcoming, the Danish "Better hEAring Rehabilitation" (BEAR) project recently developed strategies for individual hearing loss characterization and compensation. The characterization of hearing deficits is based on the concept of auditory profiling. Using various diagnostic tests, patients are stratified into four distinct groups called profiles A, B, C and D. This is achieved using a data-driven method [5]. This method was developed based on a relatively large dataset stemming from a sample of listeners with a wide range of hearing abilities who were tested with a comprehensive auditory test battery [6]. The test battery was afterwards reduced, based on considerations of cost-effectiveness and reliability, to arrive at the most informative diagnostic measures. These include loudness perception, speech intelligibility in noise, binaural hearing abilities, and spectro-temporal modulation sensitivity [7]. Furthermore, a profile-based HA fitting strategy called the BEAR strategy was proposed and evaluated in a pilot study [8], as summarized in Figure 1.

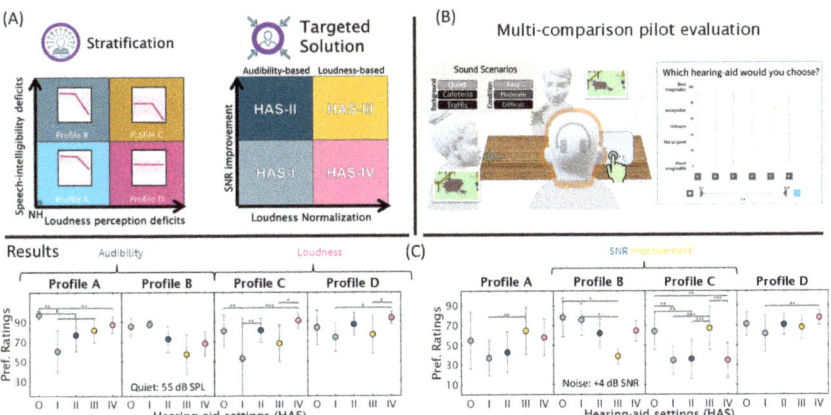

Figure 1. Overview of the pilot evaluation of the BEAR fitting strategy. (**A**) Stratification of the listeners into profiles A–D is based on two largely independent auditory dimensions, that is, speech intelligibility deficits and loudness perception deficits. Four tailored solutions (HAS I-IV) were proposed to compensate for these deficits using SNR improvement and loudness normalization, respectively. (**B**) Perceptual evaluation carried out with a HA simulator. (**C**) Results suggest that profile-C and -D listeners prefer their tailored solutions over a standard solution (HAS O), whereas profile-A and -B listeners do not show a clear preference. The image is based on the graphical abstract of [8].

Based on the results from this pilot evaluation, a large-scale randomized controlled trial was designed and carried out at two public hearing clinics. All participants underwent an initial evaluation, based on which they were stratified into one of the four auditory profiles. They were then randomly assigned to either the "BEAR" fitting strategy or a "current" fitting strategy. The participants assigned to the "current" strategy were fitted with HAs in accordance with current best clinical practice. That is, insertion gains (IGs) according to the "National Acoustic Laboratories—Non-Linear version 2" (NAL-NL2) fitting formula, which aims to maximize speech intelligibility and which was optimized based on empirical adjustments [9,10], were prescribed and verified using real-ear measurements (REM) [11]. Besides, earpieces and advanced feature settings were selected based on the recommendations made in the fitting software. In contrast, the participants assigned to the "BEAR" strategy were fitted with HAs depending on their profile membership. That is, IGs were prescribed based on the BEAR rationale [8] and verified using REM, and earpieces and advanced feature settings were chosen based on SNR improvement targets prescribed by the BEAR rationale [8].

The current report focuses on the clinical implementation of the BEAR fitting strategy. Its purpose is to demonstrate the transfer of this strategy to the hearing aids used in the large-scale clinical study. Technical measurements characterizing the HA fittings were performed in the laboratory to ensure that the targeted SNR improvement was achieved. Furthermore, REM performed in the clinics on the HA fittings made as part of the large-scale clinical study were evaluated.

2. The BEAR Rationale at a Glance

The BEAR rationale [8] includes the prescription of target gains and advanced feature settings, as summarized by the following formula:

$$\text{BEAR}(l, f, p) = 0.31 \cdot HTL(f) + \alpha(l, f, p) + \delta(p)$$

where $HTL(f)$ denotes the hearing thresholds at different frequencies, $\alpha(l, f, p)$ denotes gain correction factors applied at different input levels (l) and frequencies (f) and for the different profiles (p), and $\delta(p)$ denotes the SNR improvement to be applied for the different profiles (p). The constant factor 0.31 reflects the proportion of gain applied in relation to the HTL ("1-third rule"); for convenience, we use that specific value as it is specified in the original NAL formula [12,13]. The term $+\delta(p)$ does not represent an arithmetic sum but the SNR improvement. It does not affect the insertion gain.

To implement the BEAR rationale in three different commercially available devices, the key properties needing to be transferred first had to be identified. Table 1 summarizes the priorities chosen for the clinical implementation. To implement the BEAR rationale in three different commercially available HA devices, the key properties needing to be transferred had to be identified. Table 1 summarizes the priorities chosen for the clinical implementation. The SNR improvement was achieved by optimizing the settings of the directionality and noise reduction algorithms. The advanced features used in this study are shown in Appendix B (Table A1). Adaptive algorithms were not considered, and only features that aim for SNR improvement were activated in the BEAR fittings.

Table 1. Summary of the key properties (acoustic coupling, gain prescription, and SNR improvement) for implementing the BEAR rationale in commercially available devices.

	HA Setting	Acoustic Coupling	Gain Prescription	SNR Improvement
BEAR strategy	A	Standard or custom ear-tips (open fit)	Maximize speech audibility	Small
	B	Custom ear-molds with venting	Maximize speech audibility	Large
	C	Custom ear-molds (closed fit *)	Loudness normalization	Large
	D	Custom ear-molds (closed fit *)	Loudness normalization	Small
Current strategy	O	Same as for BEAR	NAL-NL2	Manufacturer default settings

* With small (0.6–0.8 mm) vents.

3. Challenges to the Clinical BEAR Implementation

A number of challenges related to the clinical implementation of the BEAR rationale were identified, as listed below:

- Commercial fitting tools were not suited for the implementation, as they could not readily accommodate all required HA settings.
- While REM could be used for verifying IG targets, no clinically feasible method for verifying SNR improvement targets is currently available.

- The BEAR strategy had to be sufficiently different from the current HA fitting strategy to warrant a formal investigation into its perceptual benefits.
- The HA solutions for the four auditory profiles had to be sufficiently different from each other to warrant a formal investigation into their perceptual benefits.

4. Methods

For the final implementation, the BEAR rationale was slightly modified compared to the original proposal [8]. First, the proposed compression ratios had to be adjusted to settings that were practically realizable in the fitting software of the manufacturers. Second, the gain prescription was revised, so the soft input level corresponded to 55 (instead of 50) dB SPL. This was done to reduce the influence of background noise on the corresponding REM data.

The methods described below focus on a fitting tool developed for the clinical study, the procedure used for making real-ear measurements as part of the clinical study, and SNR improvement measurements made on an acoustic mannikin in preparation for the clinical study.

4.1. Clinical Fitting Tool

A clinically feasible fitting tool was developed to allow the commercial HAs to be fitted in accordance with the BEAR rationale. First, a Microsoft Excel sheet for calculating the BEAR target gains was prepared, into which the audiologists entered the audiometric thresholds at 0.25, 0.5, 1, 2, 4, and 8 kHz together with the profile of a given patient. The Excel sheet then generated a figure that was carefully designed to resemble the visual display in the REM system used for verification purposes (Affinity 2.0, Interacoustics, Middelfart, Denmark). Using the open-source software 'OnTopReplica' [14], the calculated BEAR gains were superimposed onto the visual REM display. The fitting tool and procedure are illustrated in Figure 2.

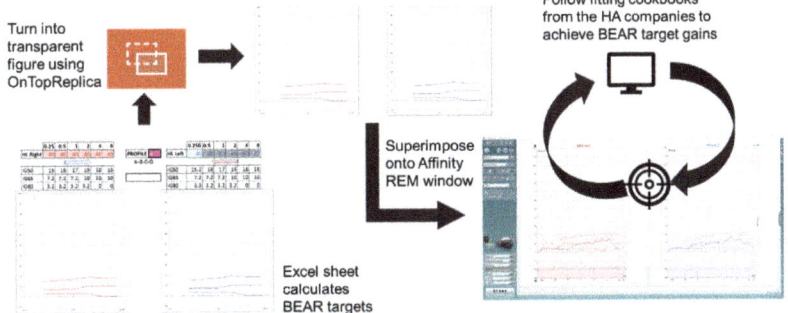

Figure 2. Illustration of the BEAR fitting tool and procedure developed for the clinical study.

The efficacy of the developed fitting tool and procedure was verified by performing several HA fittings on a CARL manikin (Ahead Simulations, Cambridge, ON, Canada). Care was taken to make the fitting process as straightforward as possible for the audiologists who handled the HA fittings in the clinical study. To accomplish this, detailed instructions were prepared to guide them through all necessary steps. Since three hearing aids from three different manufacturers were used, a set of instructions was needed for each device. Importantly, the instructions covered not only the gain adjustments, but also the activation and parameters of advanced features corresponding to the choices made for each profile in the BEAR fitting group, and the fitting protocol for the current fitting group.

4.2. Real-Ear Insertion Gain Measurements

As part of the clinical study, real-ear insertion gain (REIG) data were collected at 55, 65, and 80 dB SPL input levels to ensure close fits to the target. The International Speech Test Signal (ISTS, [15]) was used as the stimulus and played back from a loudspeaker approx. 1 m from the head of the participant. All recordings were carried out with the Interacoustics Affinity 2.0 system (Middlefart, Denmark). The REIG data were extracted as XML files and stored in an online database. Individual data files were processed to eliminate additional measurements performed during HA adjustment. Following the completion of the clinical study, information regarding the fitting strategy (current vs. BEAR) and auditory profile (A-D) was obtained and combined with the REIG data.

The participants for the clinical trial were recruited at two university hospitals (in Aalborg and Odense). Two-hundred-and-five adults with bilateral symmetric sensorineural hearing loss, Danish as their primary language, and no prior HA experience were included. They were 45–83 years old (mean and standard deviation: 68.3 ± 7.5 years), and 54% of them were male. Some participants dropped out of the study after the first visit. In total, 165 participants completed the study. At the first visit, the participants completed a clinical test battery for auditory profiling [7], based on which they were classified into a given profile. The distribution of the four auditory profiles was as follows: 53 profile-A, 92 profile-B, 14 profile-C, and 6 profile-D. There were 82 participants fitted according to the BEAR strategy and 83 participants fitted according to the current strategy. Within each profile, the distribution of the two fitting strategies was roughly equal.

4.3. SNR Improvement Measurements

To characterize the SNR improvement, electroacoustic measurements were performed in an IEC-standardized listening room at the Technical University of Denmark with a free-field setup with five loudspeakers placed in a circle with a radius of 1.5 m. At the center of the loudspeaker array, a head-and-torso simulator (HATS, type 4128, Brüel & Kjær, Nærum, Denmark) with pinnae (DZ9626-7, Brüel & Kjær, Nærum, Denmark) was placed (see Figure 3). The HATS was fitted with the test hearing devices and custom-made earpieces. The target speech signal (i.e., the ISTS) was played back from the frontal loudspeaker (0° azimuth) and so was an uncorrelated 4-talker babble noise from the other four loudspeakers (±45° and ±135° azimuth). The noise signals were calibrated to produce a sound pressure level of 70 dB SPL at the listening position.

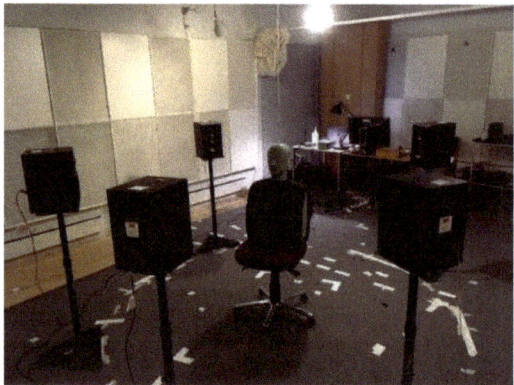

Figure 3. Picture of the test setup used for performing the SNR improvement measurements.

The measurements consisted of a series of 30 s recordings. The first 10 s of each recording were discarded. In this way, it was ensured that the advanced HA features had reached a steady state. To calculate the achieved SNR improvement, the Hagerman–Olofsson method [16] was used to separate the speech and noise signals on the HA output side. The signals from the left and right microphones were both used in the analyses by concatenating them. First, the power spectral density of the target and noise signals was estimated in 18 one-third-octave bands with center frequencies according to (ANSI S3.5-1997). The average SNR was then calculated as the difference between the power spectral density of the target and noise signals averaged across all bands.

An additional reference recording was made with the unaided HATS. The SNR improvement, ΔSNR_{avg}, was then calculated as the difference between the SNR estimated for each of the HA settings and the SNR from the unaided condition.

5. Results
5.1. REIG Measurements

Figure 4 shows mean REIGs measured at 55, 65, and 80 dB-SPL input levels. Each panel shows a comparison of the current fitting vs. one of the profile-based HA fittings (A, B, C, or D). While no differences between the two strategies are apparent for the profiles fitted according to considerations of audibility maximization (A and B), there are clear differences for the profiles fitted according to loudness normalization considerations (C and D). In both cases, the BEAR strategy provides less amplification for all input levels. This is especially clear at 80 dB SPL, where there is very little amplification below 4 kHz. Also, there are apparent gain differences between 65 and 80 dB-SPL input levels, corresponding to large compression ratios, as intended.

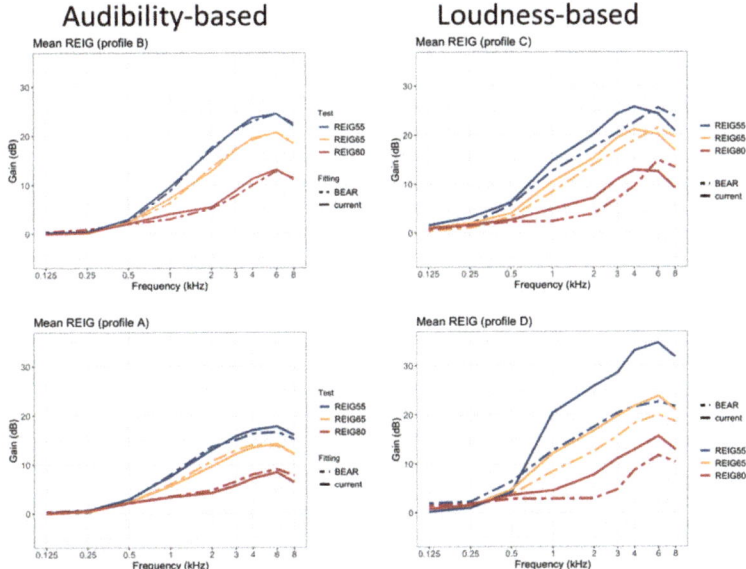

Figure 4. Mean real-ear insertion gains measured as part of the clinical study. Each panel shows data for one profile. Measurements made on participants fitted with the "current" strategy are shown with solid lines, while those made with the "BEAR" strategy are shown with dashed lines. The blue, yellow, and red lines represent input levels of 55, 65, and 80 dB SPL, respectively.

As there were only six participants in profile D, the differences in REIGs between the two fitting strategies can be largely explained based on differences in individual audiograms. To enable a comparison of the differences in gain between the two strategies for profile D, the gains measured for participants who received a BEAR fitting are compared with NAL-NL2 target gains for the same participants (i.e., for the same audiograms). This is illustrated in Appendix A. Overall, profile D is characterized by more gain at low frequencies and greater compression ratios in case of the BEAR strategy.

5.2. SNR Improvement Measurements

Figure 5 shows ΔSNR_{avg} values for three input SNRs (−5, 0, +5 dB) and the three HAs that were used in the clinical study (HA1, HA2, HA3). Each panel corresponds to one of the profiles. HA1 provided hardly any SNR improvement for profile A, but a notable SNR improvement (~3 dB) was seen for profile C. HA2 and HA3 provided 1–2 dB of SNR improvement for profiles A and D and >2 dB SNR improvement for profiles B and C. In terms of dependencies on the input SNR, there were only clear differences for profile B, especially with HA1, for which the SNR improvement decreased with increasing input SNR. This could have been a consequence of HA1 using fast-acting compression.

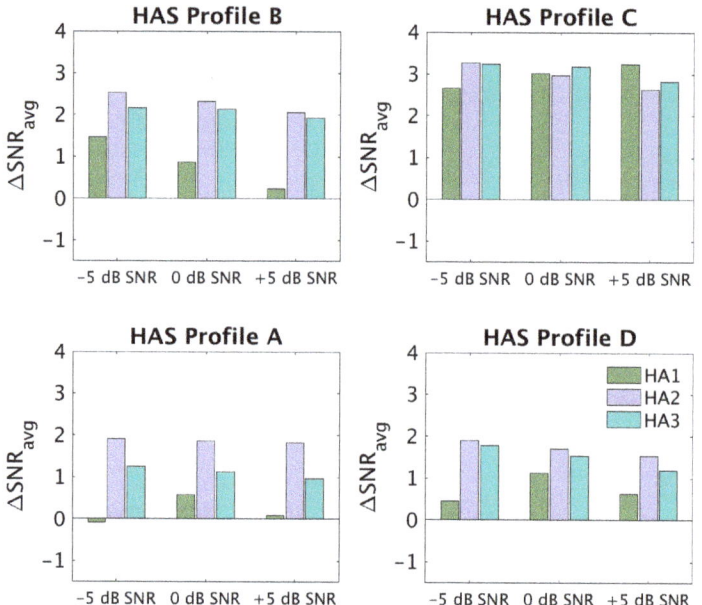

Figure 5. SNR improvement (ΔSNR_{avg}) measured at three input SNRs (−5, 0, +5 dB) for the four auditory profile-based HA fittings (A–D) and three different HAs (HA1, HA2, HA3).

6. Discussion

6.1. Differences between HA Settings for the Four BEAR Profiles

The present study focused on challenges and solutions for implementing the BEAR fitting strategy in real HAs. The results of the technical evaluation showed that the three HAs were able to provide SNR improvement targets in accordance with the BEAR strategy. This was especially true for HA1, which did not provide any SNR improvement for profiles A and D but a substantial SNR improvement for profile C and, to a lesser extent, profile B at lower input SNRs. Overall, it was therefore possible to find advanced feature settings that fulfilled the requirements.

The REIG data were collected as part of the clinical study. As expected, the IGs for HAS-A and HAS-B were very similar to the ones prescribed by NAL-NL2. This was because the BEAR rationale prescribes IG based on the same principles as NAL-NL2 (i.e., maximization of speech audibility) for these two profiles. In contrast, the IGs corresponding to HAS-C and HAS-D deviated substantially from NAL-NL2. The IGs prescribed by the BEAR rationale for HAS-C and HAS-D are based on empirical comparisons between the gains required for loudness normalization, based on loudness perception measurements. The goal here is to provide sufficient amplification to normalize loudness at soft and conversational input levels and to reduce amplification for signal inputs above 75–80 dB SPL. This is partly motivated by the expected presence of 'rollover' in profile-C listeners, which can affect speech intelligibility at above-conversational levels [17]. To achieve this compression behavior, large compression ratios are required, which are not easily achievable with commercial HAs. The reason for this limitation is that large compression ratios can compromise sound quality. Given the HAs used here, it was difficult to confirm whether the prescribed IG was normalizing the loudness as intended. A valid alternative would have been to fit the HAs while performing loudness perception tests, as suggested in [18,19], to individualize compression parameters. However, it is important to note that the profile-based HA fittings investigated here do not support the idea of using loudness normalization for all users, but only for those belonging to profiles C and D. Overall, it was possible to overcome many of the limitations in the test devices and to transfer the key properties of the BEAR rationale to them.

6.2. Limitations

A practical realization of the BEAR fitting strategy could be found based on a joint effort from the academic and industrial partners. The main limitation was that no modifications to the HA fitting software could be made. Instead, a procedure combining real-ear gain measurements with an open-source software was chosen for the gain adjustments. However, this procedure can be difficult for clinicians to perform, and thus errors can occur along the way.

While the REIG data were obtained from individual participants as part of the clinical study, the SNR improvement data could only be obtained in the laboratory. This makes a comparison of the current and BEAR fittings difficult. Currently, there is no systematic method for characterizing advanced HA signal processing in real ears. Although there are techniques that can successfully quantify signal modification [16,20], they require the use of head and torso simulators and a spatial loudspeaker configuration. Therefore, there is a need for clinically viable procedures that can be used to perform real-ear SNR measurements [21]. Ideally, it should be possible for such procedures to be routinely performed in the clinics using realistic scenarios and while the HA is operating as intended [22].

7. Conclusions

The BEAR fitting rationale was implemented for use in a large-scale clinical trial. The joint efforts by the industrial and academic partners resulted in a procedure for HA fitting that allowed the investigation of profile-based HA fittings with commercially available devices. As expected, the differences in IG between the BEAR and current fitting strategies were only apparent for profiles C and D, while the differences in SNR improvement were apparent for all profiles. The BEAR fitting rationale is the first fitting strategy that prescribes not only gain targets but also the adjustment of advanced HA features.

Author Contributions: Contributions designated as all reflect the contributions of all authors. Conceptualization; methodology; software; validation; formal analysis; and investigation, all; resources: T.D., T.N., S.S., B.K., N.B., G.R., T.P., M.B.; data curation, R.S.-L., M.W., S.K.N.; writing—original draft preparation, R.S.-L., M.W., T.N.; writing—review and editing, ALL; visualization, R.S.-L., M.W.; supervision, T.D., S.S., M.F., T.N.; project administration, T.N.; funding acquisition, T.N., T.D. All authors have read and agreed to the published version of the manuscript.

Funding: Collaboration and support by Innovationsfonden (Grand Solutions 5164-00011B), Oticon, GN Resound, WS Audiology, and other partners (University of Southern Denmark, Aalborg University, the Technical University of Denmark, Force Technology, and Aalborg, Odense and Copenhagen University Hospitals) is sincerely acknowledged.

Institutional Review Board Statement: Not applicable.

Informed Consent Statement: Informed consent was obtained from all subjects involved in the study. The study was notified to the Regional Committee on Health Research Ethics for Southern Denmark (case no. S-20162000-64).

Data Availability Statement: The data presented in this study and the BEAR protocol are available upon reasonable request from the corresponding author. The data are not publicly available due to patient data privacy. Excerpts of the data might be shared after proper anonymization.

Acknowledgments: We thank J. Zaar and S. Laugesen for their help with the SNR improvement setup and analysis. We also thank D. Hammershøi, G. Loquet, O. Cañete, R. Ordoñez, and other BEAR colleagues who provided valuable input on the BEAR procedure. We also thank colleagues from WSA, GN, and Oticon who contributed to the realization of the hearing-aid fitting guidelines.

Conflicts of Interest: The authors declare no conflict of interest.

Appendix A Comparison between BEAR and Current REIGs in Profile-D Participants

The profile-D group was relatively small. Therefore, a comparison between the REIG at 65 dB SPL and the prescribed NAL-NL2 targets is presented here. Figure A1 shows the REIGs for the three participants who were fitted according to the BEAR strategy, together with the calculated NAL-NL2 gains.

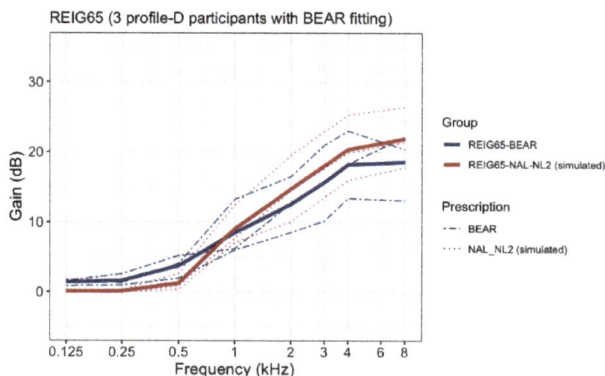

Figure A1. Mean REIGs at 65 dB SPL averaged across ears for three profile-D participants according to the BEAR strategy (blue lines). The red lines show calculated NAL-NL2 target gains.

Appendix B Hearing Devices and Advanced Features

Table A1. Settings of the advanced features for each profile-based hearing-aid fitting.

	A	B	C	D
Oticon Opn S1	Dir: Open Automatic Low transition NR simpler = 0 dB NR complex = −5 dB	Dir: Open Automatic Medium transition NR simpler = −3 dB NR complex = −7 dB	Dir: Open Automatic Very High transition NR simpler = −3 dB NR complex = −9 dB	Dir: Open Automatic Low transition NR simpler = 0 dB NR complex = −5 dB
Widex Evoke 440	Urban program. Speech and noise mode: Noise reduction comfort	Default Urban program settings	Default Impact program settings	Urban program. Speech and noise mode: Noise reduction comfort
GN Linx Quattro 9	Omni NTII: Off	Fixed Dir. NTII: Strong	Fixed Dir. NTII: Strong	Omni NTII: Off

Dir: Directionality, NR: Noise reduction; NTII: Noise Tracker II.

References

1. Grant, K.W.; Walden, B.E.; Summers, V.; Leek, M.R. Introduction: Auditory models of suprathreshold distortion in persons with impaired hearing. *J. Am. Acad. Audiol.* **2013**, *24*, 254–257. [CrossRef] [PubMed]
2. Humes, L.E.; Dubno, J.R. A Comparison of the Perceived Hearing Difficulties of Community and Clinical Samples of Older Adults. *J. Speech Lang. Hear. Res.* **2021**, *64*, 3653–3667. [CrossRef] [PubMed]

3. Kollmeier, B.; Kiessling, J. Functionality of hearing aids: State-of-the-art and future model-based solutions. *Int. J. Audiol.* **2018**, *57*, S3–S28. [CrossRef] [PubMed]
4. Vermiglio, A.J.; Soli, S.D.; Freed, D.J.; Fang, X. The Effect of Stimulus Audibility on the Relationship between Pure-Tone Average and Speech Recognition in Noise Ability. *J. Am. Acad. Audiol.* **2020**, *31*, 224–232. [CrossRef]
5. Sanchez-Lopez, R.; Fereczkowski, M.; Neher, T.; Santurette, S.; Dau, T. Robust Data-Driven Auditory Profiling Towards Precision Audiology. *Trends Hear.* **2020**, *24*, 2331216520973539. [CrossRef]
6. Sanchez-Lopez, R.; Nielsen, S.G.; El-Haj-Ali, M.; Bianchi, F.; Fereczkowski, M.; Canete, O.M.; Wu, M.; Neher, T.; Dau, T.; Santurette, S. Auditory Tests for Characterizing Hearing Deficits in Listeners With Various Hearing Abilities: The BEAR Test Battery. *Front. Neurosci.* **2021**, *15*, 724007. [CrossRef] [PubMed]
7. Sanchez-Lopez, R.; Nielsen, S.; Cañete, O.; Fereczkowski, M.; Wu, M.; Neher, T.; Dau, T.; Santurette, S. *A Clinical Test Battery for Better Hearing Rehabilitation (BEAR). Towards the Prediction of Individual AUDITORY Deficits and Hearing-Aid Benefit*; Universitätsbibliothek der RWTH Aachen: Aachen, Germany, 2019. [CrossRef]
8. Sanchez-Lopez, R.; Fereczkowski, M.; Santurette, S.; Dau, T.; Neher, T. Towards Auditory Profile-Based Hearing-Aid Fitting: Fitting Rationale and Pilot Evaluation. *Audiol. Res.* **2021**, *11*, 2. [CrossRef] [PubMed]
9. Keidser, G.; Dillon, H.; Carter, L.; O'Brien, A. NAL-NL2 empirical adjustments. *Trends Amplif.* **2012**, *16*, 211–223. [CrossRef] [PubMed]
10. Keidser, G.; Dillon, H.; Flax, M.; Ching, T.; Brewer, S. The NAL-NL2 Prescription Procedure. *Audiol. Res.* **2011**, *1*, e24. [CrossRef] [PubMed]
11. Zenker, F. Real-ear measurements by probe microphone. Definition and applications. *Auditio* **2001**, *1*, 9–14. [CrossRef]
12. Byrne, D.; Parkinson, A.; Newall, P. Hearing Aid Gain and Frequency Response Requirements for the Severely/Profoundly Hearing Impaired. *Ear Hear.* **1990**, *11*, 40–49. [CrossRef] [PubMed]
13. Byrne, D.; Tonisson, W. Selecting the Gain of Hearing Aids for Persons with Sensorineural Hearing Impairments. *Scand. Audiol.* **1976**, *5*, 51–59. [CrossRef]
14. Klopfenstein, L.C. "OnTopReplica" v3.5.1. 2018. Available online: https://github.com/LorenzCK/OnTopReplica.git (accessed on 20 August 2022).
15. Holube, I.; Fredelake, S.; Vlaming, M.; Kollmeier, B. Development and analysis of an International Speech Test Signal (ISTS). *Int. J. Audiol.* **2010**, *49*, 891–903. [CrossRef] [PubMed]
16. Hagerman, B.; Olofsson, Å. A method to measure the effect of noise reduction algorithms using simultaneous speech and noise. *Acta Acust. United Acust.* **2004**, *90*, 356–361.
17. Fereczkowski, M.; Neher, T. Predicting Aided Outcome With Aided Word Recognition Scores Measured With Linear Amplification at Above-conversational Levels. *Ear Hear.* **2022**, 10–1097. [CrossRef] [PubMed]
18. Oetting, D.; Bach, J.-H.; Krueger, M.; Vormann, M.; Schulte, M.; Meis, M. Subjective loudness ratings of vehicle noise with the hearing aid fitting methods NAL-NL2 and trueLOUDNESS. *Proc. Int. Symp. Audit. Audiol. Res.* **2019**, *7*, 289–296.
19. Oetting, D.; Hohmann, V.; Appell, J.-E.; Kollmeier, B.; Ewert, S.D. Restoring perceived loudness for listeners with hearing loss. *Ear Hear.* **2018**, *39*, 664–678. [CrossRef] [PubMed]
20. Rallapalli, V.; Anderson, M.; Kates, J.; Balmert, L.; Sirow, L.; Arehart, K.; Souza, P. Quantifying the Range of Signal Modification in Clinically Fit Hearing Aids. *Ear Hear.* **2020**, *41*, 433–441. [CrossRef] [PubMed]
21. Bell, S.L.; Creeke, S.A.; Lutman, M.E. Measuring real-ear signal-to-noise ratio: Application to directional hearing aids. *Int. J. Audiol.* **2010**, *49*, 238–246. [CrossRef] [PubMed]
22. Laugesen, S. How to compare hearing-aid processing of real speech and a speech-modified stimulus for objective validation of hearing-aid fittings? *Proc. Int. Symp. Audit. Audiol. Res.* **2020**, *7*, 317–324.

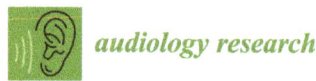

Article

Sound Quality Factors Inducing the Autonomous Sensory Meridian Response

Ryota Shimokura

Graduate School of Engineering Science, Osaka University, Room D436, 1-3 Machikaneyama, Toyonaka 560-8531, Japan; rshimo@sys.es.osaka-u.ac.jp; Tel./Fax: +81-6-6850-6376

Abstract: The acoustical characteristics of auditory triggers often recommended to generate the autonomous sensory meridian response (ASMR) on Internet platforms were investigated by parameterizing their sound qualities following Zwicker's procedure and calculating autocorrelation (ACF)/interaural cross-correlation (IACF) functions. For 20 triggers (10 human- and 10 nature-generated sounds), scores (on a five-point Likert scale) of the ASMR, perceived loudness, perceived pitch, comfort, and perceived closeness to the sound image were obtained for 26 participants by questionnaire. The results show that the human-generated sounds were more likely to trigger stronger ASMR than nature-generated sounds, and the primary psychological aspect relating to the ASMR was the perceived closeness, with the triggers perceived more closely to a listener having higher ASMR scores. The perceived closeness was evaluated by the loudness and roughness (among Zwicker's parameter) for the nature-generated sounds and the interaural cross-correlation coefficient (IACC) (among ACF/IACF parameters) for the human-generated sounds. The nature-generated sounds with higher loudness and roughness and the human-generated sounds with lower IACC were likely to evoke the ASMR sensation.

Keywords: autonomous sensory meridian response; loudness; roughness; interaural cross-correlation coefficient

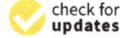

Citation: Shimokura, R. Sound Quality Factors Inducing the Autonomous Sensory Meridian Response. *Audiol. Res.* 2022, 12, 574–584. https://doi.org/10.3390/audiolres12050056

Academic Editor: Agnieszka Szczepek

Received: 25 August 2022
Accepted: 12 October 2022
Published: 13 October 2022

Publisher's Note: MDPI stays neutral with regard to jurisdictional claims in published maps and institutional affiliations.

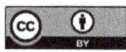

Copyright: © 2022 by the author. Licensee MDPI, Basel, Switzerland. This article is an open access article distributed under the terms and conditions of the Creative Commons Attribution (CC BY) license (https:// creativecommons.org/licenses/by/ 4.0/).

1. Introduction

The autonomous sensory meridian response (ASMR) is an atypical sensory phenomenon in which individuals experience a tingling, static sensation across the scalp and back of the neck in response to specific triggering audio and visual stimuli or to light touch [1]. This sensation is widely reported to promote relaxation, wellbeing, and sleep, and there are many ASMR-related channels on YouTube. Some researchers have examined the relationship between the ASMR and misophonia [2–4]. Misophonia is an auditory disorder of decreased tolerance to specific sounds or their associated stimuli such as oral sounds (e.g., loud breathing, chewing, swallowing), clicking sounds (e.g., keyboard tapping, finger tapping, windshield wipers), and sounds associated with movement (e.g., fidgeting) [5–8]. The ASMR triggers produce positive emotions associated with an increase of wellbeing, while the misophonia triggers produce negative emotions associated with fight-or-flight responses. Although the displayed emotions are opposite, both are caused commonly by hypersensitivities to sound triggers, and it is possible that the acoustical characteristics of the ASMR triggers may explain the occurrence mechanism of the misophonia. Actually, a previous study reported that people who experienced the ASMR were more likely to have a risk of misophonia [2].

Several common audio and visual stimuli (triggers) that induce the ASMR are known, and an online ASMR experience questionnaire completed by 475 individuals identified the trigger types as whispering (75%), personal attention (69%), crisp sounds (64%), and slow movements (53% participants reporting the ASMR experience) [1]. Following this questionnaire, many studies on the ASMR have empirically selected such highly possible triggers [9–13]. However, it is not clear which physical characteristics of these triggers induce the ASMR.

In the case of audio signals, numerical models have been proposed to define the sound quality. Perceptual characteristics of the hearing of sound are the loudness, pitch, and timbre, and the sound quality is expressed generally by numerical algorithms based on varying sound pressure. As an example, Zwicker's parameters (loudness, sharpness, roughness, and fluctuation strength) have been used to evaluate the sound quality of environmental noise [14]. The loudness is the psychological sound intensity, and it is calculated by transforming the frequency onto the Bark scale, considering the effects of frequency and temporal masking, and counting the area of the loudness pattern [15]. The loudness of a pure tone with a frequency of 1 kHz and sound pressure level of 40 dB is defined as being 1 sone. The sharpness is a measure of the sound acuity and high-frequency component, and is obtained by adding a weight function to its specific loudness [16]. The sharpness of a noise at 60 dB in a critical band at 1 kHz is defined as being 1 acum. The roughness is a fundamental hearing sensation caused by sound with rapid amplitude modulation (15–300 Hz) and is quantified on the basis of the modulation frequency and depth of the time-varying loudness [16]. The roughness of a 1 kHz tone at 60 dB with a 100% amplitude modulation (modulation depth of 1) at 70 Hz is defined as being 1 asper. The fluctuation strength is similar in principle to roughness except that it quantifies the subjective perception of the slower (up to 20 Hz) amplitude modulation of a sound, and it is calculated from the modulation frequency and depth of the time-varying loudness [16]. The fluctuation strength produced by a 1 kHz tone at 60 dB with a 100% amplitude modulated at 4 Hz is defined as being 1 vacil.

The other procedure for evaluating sound quality is using the autocorrelation and interaural cross-correlation functions (ACF and IACF) frequently used for music and acoustics in concert halls [17]. Our auditory perceptions are deeply related to the timing of nerve firings caused by binaurally detected sounds, and the ACF and IACF are modeled in the processors of the auditory nerve [18,19]. Three parameters can be calculated from ACF analyses of monoaurally recorded sound: (1) the delay time of the maximum peak (τ_1), (2) the amplitude of the first maximum peak (ϕ_1) and (3) the width of the peak at the original time [$W_{\Phi(0)}$] (see Section 2.2 for details). The fundamental frequency ($1/\tau_1$ Hz) and the pitch strength of the sound are τ_1 and ϕ_1, respectively. The spectral centroid of the original signal is $W_{\Phi(0)}$, with longer and shorter values, respectively, corresponding to lower and higher centroid values of spectral energy signals. These ACF parameters explain not only the musical motif suitable for a specific concert hall [17] but also annoyance induced by noise [20,21] and speech intelligibility [22,23]. From the IACF analyses of binaurally recorded sound, the interaural cross-correlation coefficient (IACC) can be calculated (see Section 2.1 for details). The IACC is the maximum peak amplitude of the IACF whose delay time is within ±1 ms. The IACC is related to the subjective sound diffuseness, which means that a higher IACC corresponds to the listener perceiving a well-defined direction of the incoming sound, whereas a lower IACC corresponds to a well-diffused sound. Such ACF and IACF parameters have also been used for the evaluation of several types of noise [24–27].

The present study identified physical factors that induce the auditory-based ASMR sensation using the four Zwicker parameters and four ACF/IACF parameters. We prepared a total of 20 sound motifs likely to induce the ASMR and calculated the eight sound quality parameters. To confirm the occurrence of the ASMR, previous studies have adopted physiological (e.g., functional magnetic resonance imaging or heat rate) [11,28,29] and psychological (e.g., questionaries) [1,9,10,12,13] procedures. The present study adopted the psychological approach, with participants quantifying the degree of the perceived ASMR on a five-point Likert scale. In addition to the ASMR, the participants scored four subjective sensations (subjective loudness, pitch, comfort, and closeness) at the same time. We examined the correlation of the ASMR scores with the four subjective sensations and eight sound quality parameters.

2. Method

2.1. ASMR Triggers and Sound Quality Parameters

The 10 auditory ASMR triggers (human-generated sounds) used in the study, and 10 healing sounds (nature-generated sounds) recorded binaurally were added for the comparison (Table 1). The human- and nature-generated sounds were obtained from several websites and music distribution sites, respectively. The human-generated sounds were recorded by a dummy head microphone or a binaurally wearing microphone. Although the nature-generated sounds do not have information on the recording devices, the participants of this study could perceive the sound images close to them with binaural hearing. For the sake of expediency, both sounds are called as trigger. The human- and nature-generated sounds, respectively, represent sounds generated by human behaviors (e.g., the cutting of vegetables and typing at a keyboard) and natural phenomena (e.g., waves and rain). The time length of each trigger was 50 s, and the sound energy was set at the same equivalent continuous A-weighted sound pressure level (L_{Aeq}) of 45 dBA.

Table 1 lists the sound quality parameters. The Zwicker parameters were calculated using a Matlab command embedded in Auditory Toolbox [30]. The calculation algorithms were based on work in the literature [14–16]. The calculations of roughness and fluctuation strength had running steps of 0.5 ms and 2 ms, respectively, along the time length of 50 s, and Table 1 lists average values of the time-varying parameters.

Table 1. Human- and nature-generated sounds and calculated Zwicker's and ACF/IACF parameters.

	Sound Source		Zwicker's Parameters				ACF/IACF Parameters			
	Short Title	Contents	Loudness [sone]	Sharpness [acum]	Roughness [asper]	Fluctuation Strength [vacil]	τ_1 [ms]	ϕ_1	$W_{\Phi(0)}$ [ms]	IACC
Human-generated sound	Cutting	Cutting vegetable	6.20	1.63	0.07	1.31	2.52	0.20	0.26	0.58
	Fizzwater	Stirring carbonated water	4.15	3.25	0.06	0.02	0.22	0.29	0.06	0.09
	Typing	Typing a keyboard	5.75	2.22	0.10	0.59	0.86	0.15	0.09	0.19
	Heels	Footsteps of high heels	5.58	1.58	0.05	0.43	1.56	0.19	0.36	0.37
	Book	Flipping a book	6.01	1.94	0.07	0.06	1.40	0.13	0.13	0.23
	Brush	Brushing something	6.79	1.78	0.07	0.05	1.99	0.15	0.14	0.49
	Shampoo	Washing hair with shampoo	5.67	2.33	0.08	0.33	1.92	0.04	0.10	0.05
	Hair	Cutting hair	6.34	2.17	0.01	0.39	0.93	0.42	0.09	0.33
	Pen	Writing with pen	6.08	2.54	0.01	0.39	0.42	0.29	0.06	0.29
	Earpick	Earpick	6.86	1.30	0.11	0.74	6.45	0.05	0.40	0.02
Nature-generated sound	Fire	Building a fire	7.28	1.88	0.13	0.03	3.32	0.11	0.12	0.86
	Bubble	Bubbles under water	6.23	0.70	0.06	0.07	6.74	0.21	0.77	0.40
	Brook	Murmur of a brook	5.43	1.87	0.11	0.07	1.70	0.13	0.15	0.12
	Waves	Sound of waves	5.83	1.43	0.05	0.06	3.63	0.05	0.30	0.38
	Rain	Sound of rain	5.92	2.11	0.06	0.10	3.63	0.05	0.30	0.58
	Lava	Lava flowing	5.90	2.53	0.15	0.02	0.68	0.09	0.07	0.72
	Cricket	Bell-ringing cricket	3.78	3.19	0.06	0.02	0.48	0.84	0.07	0.76
	Cicada	Evening cicada	2.77	2.69	0.02	0.02	0.28	0.95	0.09	0.93
	Volcano	Bubbles of mud volcano	7.11	1.46	0.12	0.29	1.65	0.15	0.22	0.07
	Bamboo	Wind through bamboo forest	4.98	3.13	0.07	0.06	3.76	0.02	0.06	0.26

The ACF parameters were calculated from the normalized ACF:

$$\phi_{ll}(\tau) = \phi_{ll}(\tau; s, T) = \frac{\Phi_{ll}(\tau; s, T)}{\Phi_{ll}(0; s, T)}, \quad (1)$$

where

$$\Phi_{ll}(\tau; s, T) = \frac{1}{2T} \int_{s-T}^{s+T} p_l'(t) p_l'(t+\tau) dt. \quad (2)$$

Here, τ is the delay time [s], s is the running step [s], $2T$ is the integration interval [s] and $p_l'(t)$ is the sound in the left channel at time t after passing through an A-weighted network. The ACF parameters were the (1) delay time of the maximum peak (τ_1), (2) amplitude of the first maximum peak (ϕ_1) and (3) width of the peak at $\tau = 0$ ($W_{\Phi(0)}$), calculated by doubling the delay time at which the normalized ACF becomes 0.5 times that at the origin of the delay (Figure 1a). Additionally, τ_1 and ϕ_1 are related to the pitch (high or low) and pitch strength (clear or ambiguous) perceived in the periodical part of the sound. The spectral centroid is equivalent to $W_{\Phi(0)}$, and a sound with greater $W_{\Phi(0)}$ is thus perceived as having a lower pitch in the noisy part.

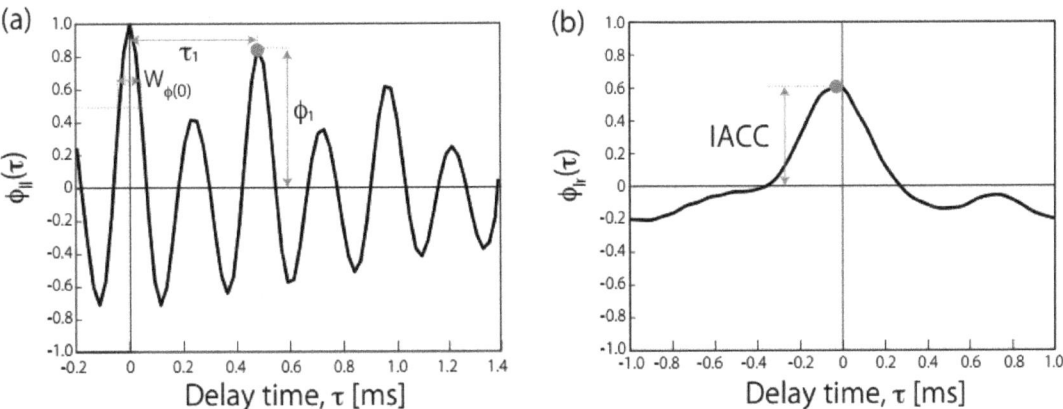

Figure 1. (a) Normalized ACF of *Cicada* as a nature-generated sound and (b) normalized IACF of *Cutting* as a human-generated sound. The definitions of τ_1, ϕ_1, $W_{\Phi(0)}$ and the IACC are included.

The IACC was calculated from the normalized IACF:

$$\phi_{lr}(\tau) = \phi_{lr}(\tau) = \frac{\Phi_{lr}(\tau; s, T)}{\sqrt{\Phi_{ll}(0; s, T) \Phi_{rr}(0; s, T)}}, \quad (3)$$

where

$$\Phi_{lr} = \frac{1}{2T} \int_{s-T}^{s+T} p_l'(t) p_r'(t+\tau) dt. \quad (4)$$

Here, Φ_{rr} is the ACF for the right channel and $p_r'(t)$ is the A-weighted sound in the right channel. The IACC is the maximum peak amplitude of the IACF whose delay time is within ±1 ms (Figure 1b). The IACC is related to the subjective sound diffuseness mentioned in the Introduction. The integration interval ($2T$) and running step (s) were, respectively, 1 and 0.5 s for the both ACF and IACF calculations, and Table 1 lists average values of the time-varying parameters.

2.2. Participants

We recruited 26 participants (20 men and 6 women; age: 21.7 ± 0.4 years) who had normal hearing. All participants self-reported that they knew of the ASMR through watching Japanese YouTube channels. The institutional ethics committee approved the experimental protocol (approval code: R3-19).

2.3. Tasks and Procedures

After listening to the ASMR trigger (50 s) through headphones (HD598, Sennheiser, Wedemark, Germany) binaurally, the participants were instructed to provide scores on a five-point Likert scale in the subsequent 10 s. The L_{Aeq} at the ear positions was adjusted to 45 dBA. After mounting the headphones on a head and torso simulator (type 4128; Brüel & Kjær, Naerum, Denmark), the output level was adjusted to the 45 dBA in the average of the left and right channels. The participants were asked to give scores (−2, −1, 0, 1 or 2) for the degree of perceived loudness (from −2: not so loud to 2: very loud), perceived pitch (from −2: very low to 2: very high), comfort (from −2: not so comfortable to 2: very comfortable), perceived closeness to the sound image (from −2: very far to 2: very close) and ASMR (from −2: not feeling an ASMR to 2: feeling a strong ASMR) on the question sheet. The order of presentation of the AMSR triggers was randomized. The experiment was conducted in an anechoic chamber (L_{Aeq} of the background noise below 30 dB) at Osaka University, Japan. The Matlab was used to calculate the statistical values in the following section.

3. Results

Figure 2 shows the average scores of the subjective loudness, pitch, comfort, closeness, and ASMR for the human- (black symbols) and nature-generated (gray symbols) sounds. The subjective loudness, closeness, and ASMR scores tended to be higher for the human-generated sounds than for the nature-generated sounds. According to a *t*-test of the total scores of the human- (260 = 10 ASMR triggers × 26 participants) and nature-generated (260) sounds, there were significant differences in the subjective loudness (t_{338} = 3.65, $p < 0.01$), closeness (t_{338} = 8.69, $p < 0.01$), and ASMR (t_{338} = 7.84, $p < 0.01$). In contrast, the comfort was higher for the nature-generated sounds (t_{338} = 6.28, $p < 0.01$) and there was no significant difference in the perceived pitch between the nature- and human-generated sounds (t_{338} = 0.28, $p = 0.78$). The three sounds with the highest ASMR values were Earpick, Shampoo, and Book for the human-generated sounds and Volcano, Lava, and Bubble for the nature-generated sounds, and they were commonly perceived to be close. The three sounds with the lowest ASMR values were Cutting, Heels, and Brush for the human-generated sound and Cicada, Bamboo, and Rain for the nature-generated sounds, and they were commonly perceived to be far.

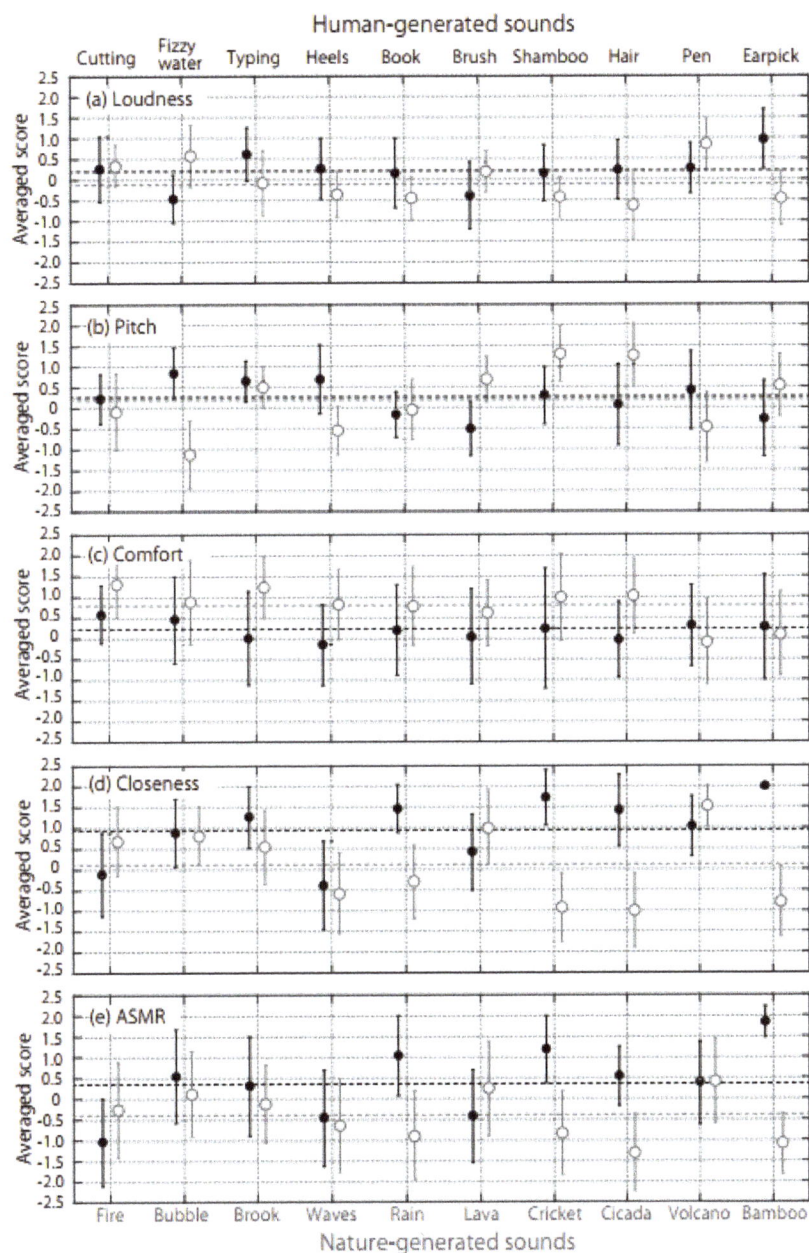

Figure 2. Average scores for (**a**) loudness, (**b**) pitch, (**c**) comfort, (**d**) closeness, and (**e**) the ASMR. Black and gray symbols are results for human- and nature-generated sounds, respectively. The bar on each symbol shows standard deviations. The black and gray horizontal dot lines are total averaged scores for human- and nature-generated sounds, respectively.

Table 2 shows the Pearson correlation coefficients of the ASMR scores with the sound quality parameters that had normal distributions. The ASMR scores of the nature-generated sounds were strongly correlated with loudness and roughness among the Zwicker parameters. Meanwhile, the ASMR scores of the human-generated sounds were strongly correlated with the IACC among the ACF/IACF parameters. Figure 3 shows the ASMR scores as functions of loudness, roughness, and IACC which showed high Pearson correlation coefficients. The strong negative relationship could be observed in the IACC for the human-generated sounds, while the positive relationships could be observed in the loudness and roughness for the nature-generated sounds. Table 2 lists the correlation coefficients of the ASMR scores with the scores of the other psychological judgements, too. The subjective loudness had a high correlation with the ASMR generated by the nature-generated sounds. Additionally, closeness had a high correlation with the ASMR generated by both human- and nature-generated sounds.

Table 2. Correlation coefficients of the ASMR scores among Zwicker's parameters, ACF/IACF parameters and subjective judgements (**: $p < 0.01$, *: $p < 0.05$).

	Zwicker's Parameters				ACF/IACF Parameters				Subjective Judgements			
	Loudness	Sharpness	Roughness	Fluctuation Strength	τ_1	Φ_1	$W_{\Phi(0)}$	IACC	Subjective Loudness	Pitch	Comfort	Closeness
ASMR (Total)	0.42	−0.21	0.27	0.15	0.12	−0.36	0.06	−0.67 **	0.64 **	−0.29	−0.38	0.93 **
ASMR (Human)	0.04	0.11	0.32	−0.30	0.39	−0.32	−0.04	−0.89 **	0.38	−0.20	0.02	0.93 **
ASMR (Nature)	0.73 *	−0.61	0.77 **	0.47	0.14	−0.46	0.34	−0.41	0.92 **	−0.53	−0.17	0.96 **

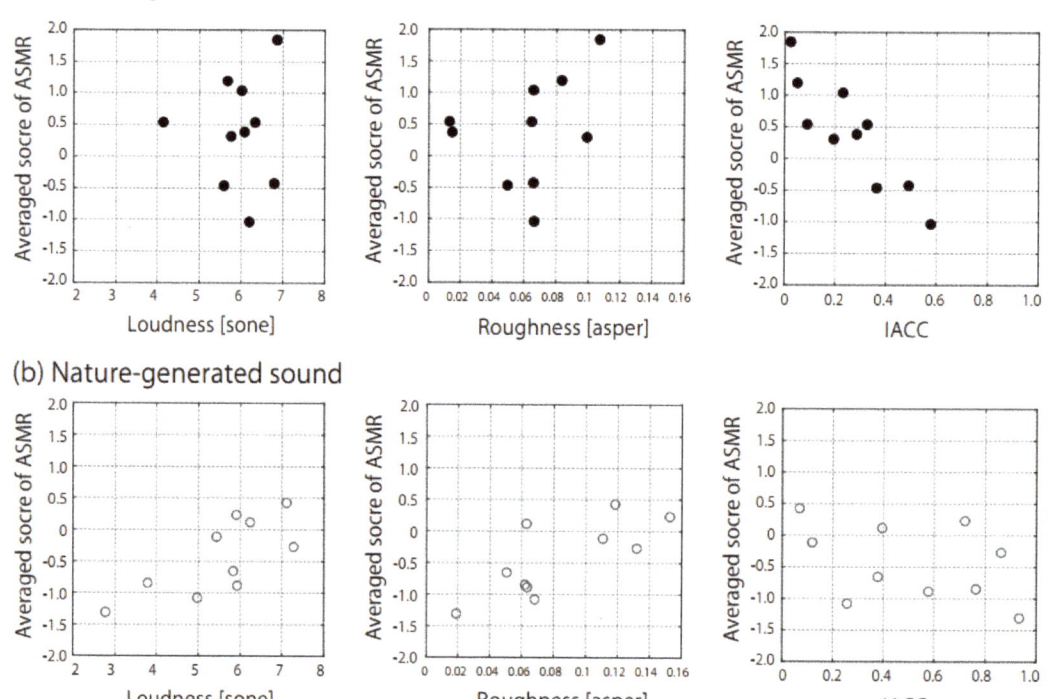

Figure 3. Relationships of the ASMR scores with loudness, roughness, and IACC for (**a**) human-generated sounds (black symbols) and (**b**) nature-generated sounds (gray symbols).

4. Discussion

The primary reason why the ASMR scores of the human-generated sounds were significantly higher than the nature-generated sounds may be the distance from the sound source to the receiver. In fact, the perceived closeness was strongly related to the ASMR sensation (Table 2). The human-generated sounds were recorded at a position close to the binaural devices whereas the nature-generated sounds were recorded at a certain distance from the sound source. Additionally, the ASMR triggers used in previous studies (e.g., whisper voice, personal attention, and crisp sounds) were recorded close to the binaural microphone [1,9–13]. In these triggers, the personal attention refers to role-play videos that concentrate on the viewer, so that it is not just an ASMR trigger but the scenario/context in which the triggers occur. To examine acoustical aspects in the triggers, sounds including the scenario/context (e.g., speech) were removed from the triggers used in this study. However, the Earpick, Shampoo, and Hair sounds that had high ASMR scores made the participants imagine to be acted upon themselves. It seems undeniable that such unintended personal attention might help the ASMR sensations for these triggers, and the very closed triggers to the participants are likely to induce the pseudo-personal attention.

For nature-generated sounds, sound qualities relating to higher loudness and roughness induced the ASMR experience (Figure 3). These parameters also had high correlations with the closeness scores (loudness: $r = 0.73$, $p < 0.05$, roughness: $r = 0.77$, $p < 0.01$). The nearby sounds produce the ASMR, whereas some listeners are annoyed by sounds close to their ears. Therefore, the comfort scores were significantly lower for the human-generated sounds (Figure 2c). Although it is well known that people who experience ASMRs report feeling relaxed and sleepy after watching and listening to ASMR content, some people feel annoyance from the triggers [4]. The hypersensitivity for the auditory perception is the same origin for the ASMR and misophonia; however, higher-order cognitive processing may divide expressed emotions into the preference for the ASMR or annoyance for the misophonia [3]. The very closed sound makes the listeners imagine either the positive personal attention or negative invasion of territory. Separation at the cognitive processing may be related to the different interpretation of the closeness. If this study contains speech signals addressing the participants, the comfort scores for the human-generated sounds may be improved.

Although a previous ASMR study reported that sounds with a lower pitch were more likely to produce an intense ASMR sensation [9], the pitch scores and ACF/IACF parameters relating to pitch (i.e., τ_1, ϕ_1 and $W_{\Phi(0)}$) did not affect the ASMR score (Figure 2b and Table 2). The bass or low-frequency response is higher when a sound source is close to a directional or cardioid microphone (in what is known as the acoustical proximity effect) [31]. In this study, the acoustical proximity effect might occur to the same degree for any human-generated sound that is sufficiently close to the binaural microphones.

The human-generated sounds with a lower IACC produced a stronger ASMR sensation (Figure 3). The IACC is related to the spatial characteristics of a sound field, and it can thus control the location of a sound image. In concert halls (having a diffused sound field), the IACC is lower when the distance between the sound source and receiver is greater [32], because the direct sound that tends to increase the IACC is weakened relative to reflections and reverberations. In contrast, in laboratory experiments, the IACC can be controlled by changing the interchannel phase difference of stereo loudspeakers in front of the listener, and a sound with lower IACC can generate a sound image closer to the listener (in what is referred to as auditory distance rendering) [33–37]. This phenomenon observed in auditory distance rendering agrees with the results of the present study. However, the binaural phase of the ASMR triggers used in this study was not manipulated digitally; therefore, there may be another explanation in this case. The IACC indicates the similarity of time-varied sounds entering the left and right ears. It is thus expected that sound near one ear (e.g., the sound heard when using an earpick) has low similarity (low IACC) between the ears, and we thus have to separate the relationships between the IACC and the distance from the sound image into near and far fields centering around the listener's head.

Finally, we discuss the possible applications of these findings in clinical treatments for misophonia. The most successfully used treatment at the clinical scene is cognitive behavioral therapy (CBT) [38–42]. The CBT protocol constitutes four different techniques: task concentration exercises, counterconditioning, stimulus manipulation, and relaxation exercises. Following treatment, 48% of the patients showed a significant reduction of misophonia symptoms [43]. In a session of stimulus manipulation, the patients are instructed to change the pitch and time interval of sound triggers by using an audio-editing software, and this manipulation initiates a sense of control over their personal misophonic trigger sounds. In this study, the IACC is the most effective factor to control the ASMR sensation, so the change of IACC (e.g., convolution with binaural impulse responses) may be effective to let the patients know the misophonic trigger sounds under their control.

5. Conclusions

The following conclusions are drawn from the results of the study.

(1) Human-generated sounds are more likely to trigger stronger ASMRs than nature-generated sounds.
(2) Among possible ASMR auditory triggers, sounds perceived to be close to the listener are more likely to evoke the ASMR sensation.
(3) In the case of nature-generated sounds, the ASMR triggers with higher loudness and roughness among Zwicker parameters are more likely to evoke the ASMR sensation.
(4) In the case of human-generated sounds, the ASMR triggers with a lower IACC among the ACF/IACF parameters are more likely to evoke the ASMR sensation.

Funding: This research was supported by a Grant-in-Aid for Science Research (B) from the Japan Society for the Promotion of Science (18H03560).

Institutional Review Board Statement: The institutional ethics committee in Osaka University approved the experimental protocol (approval code: R3-19).

Informed Consent Statement: Informed consent was obtained from all subjects involved in the study. Written informed consent has been obtained from the patients to publish this paper.

Data Availability Statement: Not applicable.

Acknowledgments: The author thanks the participants for their cooperation during the experiment, Yoshiki Konosu for helping with the experiment.

Conflicts of Interest: The authors declare no conflict of interest.

References

1. Barratt, E.L.; Davis, N.J. Autonomous Sensory Meridian Response (ASMR): A flow-like mental state. *PeerJ* **2015**, *3*, e851. [CrossRef] [PubMed]
2. McErlean, A.B.J.; Banissy, M.J. Increased misophonia in self-reported Autonomous Sensory Meridian Response. *PeerJ* **2018**, *6*, e5351. [CrossRef] [PubMed]
3. McGeoch, P.D.; Rouw, R. How everyday sounds can trigger strong emotion: ASMR, misophonia and the feeling of wellbeing. *BioEssays.* **2020**, *42*, 2000099. [CrossRef] [PubMed]
4. Tada, K.; Hasegawa, R.; Kondo, H. Sensitivity to everyday sounds: ASMR, misophonia, and autistic traits. *Jpn. J. Psychol.* **2022**, *93*, 263–269. [CrossRef]
5. Jastreboff, M.M.; Jastreboff, P.J. Components of decreased sound tolerance: Hyperacusis, misophonia, phonophobia. *ITHS News Lett.* **2001**, *2*, 5–7.
6. Jastreboff, P.J.; Jastreboff, M.M. Treatments for decreased sound tolerance (hyperacusis and misophonia). In *Seminars in Hearing*; Thieme Medical Publishers: New York, NY, USA, 2014; Volume 35, pp. 105–120.
7. Møller, A.R. Misophonia, phonophobia, and 'exploding head' syndrome. In *Textbook of Tinnitus*; Møller, A.R., Langguth, B., DeRidder, D., Kleinjung, T., Eds.; Springer: New York, NY, USA, 2011; pp. 25–27.
8. Wu, M.S.; Lewin, A.B.; Murphy, T.K.; Storch, E.A. Misophonia: Incidence, phenomenology, and clinical correlates in an undergraduate student sample. *J. Clin. Psychol.* **2014**, *70*, 994–1007. [CrossRef]
9. Barratt, E.L.; Spence, C.; Davis, N.J. Sensory determinants of the autonomous sensory meridian response (ASMR): Understanding the triggers. *PeerJ.* **2017**, *5*, e3846. [CrossRef]

10. Fredborg, B.; Clark, J.; Smith, S.D. An examination of personality traits associated with autonomous sensory meridian response (ASMR). *Front. Psychol.* **2017**, *8*, 247. [CrossRef]
11. Poerio, G.L.; Blakey, E.; Hostler, T.J.; Veltri, T. More than a feeling: Autonomous sensory meridian response (ASMR) in characterized by reliable changes in affect and physiology. *PLoS ONE* **2018**, *13*, e0196645. [CrossRef]
12. Smith, S.D.; Fredborg, B.; Kornelsen, J. Functional connectivity associated with different categories of autonomous sensory meridian response (ASMR) triggers. *Conscious. Cogn.* **2020**, *85*, 103021. [CrossRef]
13. Swart, T.R.; Bowling, N.C.; Banissy, M.J. ASMR-experience questionnaire (AEQ): A data-driven step towards accurately classifying ASMR responders. *Br. J. Psychol.* **2022**, *113*, 68–83. [CrossRef]
14. Zwicker, E.; Fastl, H. *Psychoacoustics: Facts and Models*; Springer: Berlin/Heidelberg, Germany, 1999.
15. *ISO 532-1*; Acoustics—Methods for Calculating Loudness—Part 1: Zwicker Method. International Organization for Standardization: Geneva, Switzerland, 2017.
16. *DIN 45692*; Measurement Technique for the Simulation of the Auditory Sensation of Sharpness. German Institute for Standardization: Berlin, Germany, 2009.
17. Ando, Y. 5. Prediction of subjective preference in concert halls. In *Concert Hall Acoustics*; Springer: Berlin/Heidelberg, Germany, 1995; pp. 70–88.
18. Cariani, P.A.; Delgutte, B. Neural correlates of the pitch of complex tones. I. Pitch and pitch salience. *J. Neurophysiol.* **1996**, *76*, 1698–1716. [CrossRef] [PubMed]
19. Cariani, P.A.; Delgutte, B. Neural correlates of the pitch of complex tones. II. Pitch shift, pitch ambiguity, phase invariance, pitch circularity, rate pitch, and the dominance. *J. Neurophysiol.* **1996**, *76*, 1717–1734. [CrossRef] [PubMed]
20. Sato, S.; You, J.; Jeon, J.Y. Sound quality characteristics of refrigerator noise in real living environments with relation to psychoacoustical and autocorrelation function parameters. *J. Acoust. Soc. Am.* **2007**, *122*, 314–325. [CrossRef] [PubMed]
21. Soeta, Y.; Shimokura, R. Sound quality evaluation of air-conditioner noise based on factors of the autocorrelation function. *Appl. Acoust.* **2017**, *124*, 11–19. [CrossRef]
22. Ando, Y. Autocorrelation-based features for speech representation. *Acta Acust. United Acust.* **2015**, *101*, 145–154. [CrossRef]
23. Shimokura, R.; Akasaka, S.; Nishimura, T.; Hosoi, H.; Matsui, T. Autocorrelation factors and intelligibility of Japanese monosyllables in individuals with sensorineural hearing loss. *J. Acoust. Soc. Am.* **2017**, *141*, 1065. [CrossRef]
24. Kitamura, T.; Shimokura, R.; Sato, S.; Ando, Y. Measurement of temporal and spatial factors of a flushing toilet noise in a downstairs bedroom. *J. Temp. Des. Archit. Environ.* **2002**, *2*, 13–19.
25. Fujii, K.; Soeta, Y.; Ando, Y. Acoustical properties of aircraft noise measured by temporal and spatial factors. *J. Sound Vib.* **2001**, *241*, 69–78. [CrossRef]
26. Fujii, K.; Atagi, J.; Ando, Y. Temporal and spatial factors of traffic noise and its annoyance. *J. Temp. Des. Archit. Environ.* **2002**, *2*, 33–41.
27. Soeta, Y.; Shimokura, R. Survey of interior noise characteristics in various types of trains. *Appl. Acoust.* **2013**, *74*, 1160–1166. [CrossRef]
28. Smith, S.D.; Fredborg, B.K.; Kornelsen, J. An examination of the default mode network in individuals with autonomous sensory meridian response (AMSR). *Soc. Neurosci.* **2017**, *12*, 361–365. [CrossRef] [PubMed]
29. Lochte, B.C.; Guillory, S.A.; Richard, C.A.H.; Kelly, W.M. An fMRI investigation of neural correlates underlying the autonomous sensory median response (ASMR). *BioImpacts* **2018**, *8*, 295–304. [CrossRef]
30. Audio Toolbox. Available online: https://jp.mathworks.com/help/audio/index.html?s_tid=CRUX_lftnav (accessed on 23 September 2022).
31. Nikolov, M.E.; Blagoeva, M.E. Proximity effect frequency characteristics of directional microphones. In Proceedings of the Audio Engineering Society Convention 108, Paris, French, 19–22 February 2000.
32. Fujii, K.; Hotehama, T.; Kato, K.; Shimokura, R.; Okamoto, Y.; Suzumura, Y.; Ando, Y. Spatial distribution of acoustical parameters in concert halls: Comparison of different scattered reflections. *J. Temp. Des. Archit. Environ.* **2004**, *4*, 59–68.
33. Kurozumi, K.; Ohgushi, K. The relationship between the cross correlation coefficient of two-channel acoustic signals and sound image quality. *J. Acoust. Soc. Am.* **1983**, *74*, 1726–1733. [CrossRef]
34. Gerzon, M.A. Signal processing for simulating realistic stereo images. In Proceedings of the Audio Engineering Society Convention 93, San Francisco, CA, USA, 1–4 October 1992.
35. Kendall, G.S. The decorrelation of audio signals and its impact on spatial imagery. *Comput. Music J.* **1995**, *19*, 71–87. [CrossRef]
36. Koyama, S.; Furuya, K.; Hiwasaki, Y.; Haneda, Y. Reproducing virtual sound sources in front of a loudspeaker array using inverse wave propagator. *IEEE Trans. Audio Speech Lang. Process.* **2012**, *20*, 1746–1758. [CrossRef]
37. Jeon, S.W.; Park, Y.C.; Youn, D.H. Auditory distance rendering based on ICPD control for stereophonic 3D audio system. *IEEE Signal Process. Lett.* **2015**, *22*, 529–533. [CrossRef]
38. Bernstein, R.E.; Angell, K.L.; Dehle, C.M. A brief course of cognitive behavioral therapy for the treatment of misophonia: A case example. *Cogn. Behav. Ther.* **2013**, *6*, e10. [CrossRef]
39. Dozier, T.H. Counterconditioning treatment for misophonia. *Clin. Case Stud.* **2015**, *14*, 374–387. [CrossRef]
40. Dozier, T.H. Treating the initial physical reflex of misophonia with the neural repatterning technique: A counterconditioning procedure. *Psychol. Thought* **2015**, *8*, 189–210. [CrossRef]

41. McGuire, J.F.; Wu, M.S.; Storch, E.A. Cognitive-behavioral therapy for 2 youths with Misophonia. *J. Clin. Psychiatry* **2015**, *76*, 573–574. [CrossRef] [PubMed]
42. Reid, A.M.; Guzick, A.G.; Gernand, A.; Olsen, B. Intensive cognitive-behavioral therapy for comorbid misophonic and obsessive-compulsive symptoms: A systematic case study. *J. Obsessive Compuls. Relat. Disord.* **2016**, *10*, 1–9. [CrossRef]
43. Schröder, A.E.; Vulink, N.C.; van Loon, A.J.; Denys, D.A. Cognitive behavioral therapy is effective in misophonia: An open trial. *J. Affect. Disord.* **2017**, *217*, 289–294. [CrossRef] [PubMed]

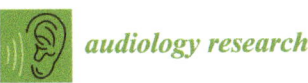

Article

Lateralization Pattern of the Weber Tuning Fork Test in Longstanding Unilateral Profound Hearing Loss: Implications for Cochlear Implantation

Mohamed Bassiouni [1,*], Sophia Marie Häußler [2], Stefan Gräbel [1], Agnieszka J. Szczepek [1] and Heidi Olze [1]

1 Corporate Member of Freie Universität Berlin, Berlin Institute of Health, Charitéplatz 1, Humboldt-Universität zu Berlin, 10117 Berlin, Germany; stefan.graebel@charite.de (S.G.); agnes.szczepek@charite.de (A.J.S.); heidi.olze@charite.de (H.O.)
2 Department of Otorhinolaryngology, University Medical Center Hamburg-Eppendorf, Martinistraße 52, 20246 Hamburg, Germany; s.haeussler@uke.de
* Correspondence: mohamed.bassiouni@charite.de; Tel.: +49-30-450-555-072

Abstract: The Weber tuning fork test is a standard otologic examination tool in patients with unilateral hearing loss. Sound should typically lateralize to the contralateral side in unilateral sensorineural hearing loss. The observation that the Weber test does not lateralize in some patients with longstanding unilateral deafness has been previously described but remains poorly understood. In the present study, we conducted a retrospective analysis of the medical records of patients with unilateral profound hearing loss (single-sided deafness or asymmetric hearing loss) for at least ten years. In this patient cohort, childhood-onset unilateral profound hearing loss was significantly associated with the lack of lateralization of the Weber tuning fork test (Fisher's exact test, $p < 0.05$) and the absence of tinnitus in the affected ear (Fisher's exact test, $p < 0.001$). The findings may imply a central adaptation process due to chronic unilateral auditory deprivation starting before the critical period of auditory maturation. This notion may partially explain the poor outcome of adult cochlear implantation in longstanding single-sided deafness. The findings may suggest a role for the Weber test as a simple, quick, and economical tool for screening poor cochlear implant candidates, thus potentially supporting the decision-making and counseling of patients with longstanding single-sided deafness.

Keywords: hearing loss; tuning fork; audiometry; single-sided deafness; tinnitus

Citation: Bassiouni, M.; Häußler, S.M.; Gräbel, S.; Szczepek, A.J.; Olze, H. Lateralization Pattern of the Weber Tuning Fork Test in Longstanding Unilateral Profound Hearing Loss: Implications for Cochlear Implantation. *Audiol. Res.* 2022, 12, 347–356. https://doi.org/10.3390/audiolres12040036

Academic Editor: Andrea Ciorba

Received: 22 May 2022
Accepted: 15 June 2022
Published: 21 June 2022

Publisher's Note: MDPI stays neutral with regard to jurisdictional claims in published maps and institutional affiliations.

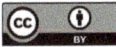

Copyright: © 2022 by the authors. Licensee MDPI, Basel, Switzerland. This article is an open access article distributed under the terms and conditions of the Creative Commons Attribution (CC BY) license (https://creativecommons.org/licenses/by/4.0/).

1. Introduction

Tuning fork tests have remained a mainstay of otologic examination for over a century. The Weber tuning fork test has been mainly used in patients with unilateral hearing loss to distinguish between sensorineural and conductive hearing loss [1–4]. In patients with conductive hearing loss, the sound should typically lateralize to the affected side, whereas in sensorineural hearing loss, it lateralizes to the contralateral side. The mechanism of sound lateralization of the Weber test has intrigued hearing health professionals for many decades [1–4]. Clinical and animal experiments have shown that bone conduction stimulates the cochlea mainly through two routes: (1) through the vibration of the middle ear ossicles and (2) vibrations of the skull itself (mainly of the cerebrospinal fluid) [4]. In the case of unilateral sensorineural hearing loss, the intercochlear intensity and phase differences lead to vibrations being perceived louder in the contralateral unaffected ear, producing sound lateralization. The observation that some patients with longstanding unilateral deafness fail to lateralize on the Weber test has been previously mentioned in the literature but remains poorly understood [2,5,6]. To date, there is no explanation as to why some patients with longstanding single-sided deafness lateralize and others do not. This article reports on thirteen cases of patients with longstanding unilateral profound hearing loss of various etiologies. These patients had different lateralization patterns on the Weber tuning fork test, seemingly related to the age of onset of deafness.

2. Materials and Methods

The study was approved by the ethics committee of Charité Medical University (approval number EA1/015/21). The analysis involved the retrospective review of the hospital records and audiograms of adult patients with profound unilateral hearing loss (UHL) of at least ten years' duration who presented to our outpatient department and/or auditory implant clinic between 2018 and 2021. Pure tone audiograms (PTA) determined the ipsilateral and contralateral hearing status. Profound hearing loss was defined by a pure tone threshold average of 90 dB or higher, as described previously [7,8]. The pure tone threshold average was considered the average threshold at four frequencies: 0.5, 1, 2, and 4 kHz. The Weber tuning fork test was performed using a standard 512 Hz tuning fork for all patients. To meet the inclusion criteria, the patients had to have an audiometric interaural asymmetry of at least 50 dB at the frequency of the tuning fork tone (512 kHz). According to the status of the contralateral ear, the patients were divided into single-sided deafness (SSD) or asymmetric hearing loss (AHL) groups. SSD was defined by contralateral a PTA four-frequency average threshold below or equal to 30 dB, while AHL was defined by a PTA four-frequency average threshold above 30dB [9,10]. Statistical analysis was performed using JMP 15 Software (Statistical Analysis Systems "SAS" Institute, Cary, NC, USA).

3. Results

3.1. Patient Cohort

Thirteen adult patients met the inclusion criteria. Their age ranged from 26 to 78 years (median 54 ± 16.3 years); seven patients were male, and six were female. All patients were diagnosed with profound unilateral hearing loss (UHL) of at least ten years' duration. The patients' epidemiological, clinical, and medical history details are summarized in Table 1. Of the 13 patients, 8 had childhood-onset UHL and 5 had adult-onset UHL. The duration of UHL ranged from 10 to 73 years. According to the status of the contralateral ear, ten patients had single-sided deafness (SSD), while three patients had asymmetric hearing loss (AHL). Eight of thirteen patients reported having tinnitus in the poorer hearing ear.

Table 1. Patient characteristics of the study cohort. AHL: asymmetric hearing loss; SSD: single-sided deafness; UHL: unilateral profound hearing loss. SSNHL: sudden sensorineural hearing loss. F: female; M: male.

	Age (Years)	Gender	Weber Test	Residual Hearing	SSD vs. AHL	Etiology	Age of Onset (Years)	Onset Classification	Duration of UHL (Years)	Tinnitus
#1	78	F	No lateralization	Yes	AHL	Infectious (scarlet fever)	6	Childhood onset	72	No
#2	34	M	Lateralized	No	SSD	Infectious (meningitis)	4	Childhood onset	30	No
#3	75	F	Lateralized	No	AHL	Surgery	22	Adult onset	53	Yes
#4	54	M	Lateralized	No	SSD	Surgery	37	Adult onset	17	Yes
#5	54	M	No lateralization	Yes	SSD	Trauma	7	Childhood onset	47	No
#6	54	M	No lateralization	No	SSD	Infectious (labyrinthitis)	4	Childhood onset	50	No
#7	56	F	No lateralization	Yes	SSD	SSNHL	46	Adult onset	10	Yes
#8	36	F	No lateralization	No	SSD	Congenital	0	Childhood onset	36	No
#9	54	M	No lateralization	No	SSD	Congenital	0	Childhood onset	54	No
#10	51	M	Lateralized	Yes	SSD	Menière's disease	33	Adult onset	18	Yes

Table 1. Cont.

	Age (Years)	Gender	Weber Test	Residual Hearing	SSD vs. AHL	Etiology	Age of Onset (Years)	Onset Classification	Duration of UHL (Years)	Tinnitus
#11	44	F	Lateralized	Yes	SSD	SSNHL	22	Adult onset	22	Yes
#12	26	F	No lateralization	No	SSD	Infectious (mumps)	3	Childhood onset	23	No
#13	78	F	No lateralization	Yes	AHL	Infectious	5	Childhood onset	73	No

3.2. Weber Test Lateralization Pattern and the Age of Onset

All but one patient with childhood-onset UHL (seven of eight patients) reported hearing the tuning fork tone during the Weber test but without lateralization to one side. In contrast, all but one patient with adult-onset UHL (four of five patients) reported lateralization to the contralateral side, and no patients lateralized to the ipsilateral side in this cohort. A contingency analysis showed a significant correlation between the age of onset (adult vs. childhood) and the pattern of lateralization of the Weber test (Fisher's exact test, $p = 0.0319$). The patients' age, gender, and duration of UHL did not significantly correlate with the Weber test result in this cohort.

Concerning tinnitus, 5 of 13 patients (38%) reported having tinnitus in the worse hearing ear (ipsilesional tinnitus). No patients with childhood-onset UHL reported having tinnitus, while all patients with adult-onset UHL reported having ipsilesional tinnitus. On a statistical contingency analysis, the absence of tinnitus correlated significantly with the lack of lateralization during the Weber test (Fisher's exact test, $p = 0.0008$). Other factors such as the ipsilateral residual hearing or the contralateral hearing status were not significantly associated with the Weber test lateralization pattern in this patient cohort.

3.3. Case Presentations (Selected Cases)

Patient #1: 78-year-old woman who suffered from scarlet fever during childhood (around the age of six), resulting in a profound hearing loss on the right side. The patient reported having heard no sounds in the right ear since childhood, even in very noisy environments. The patient also denied having tinnitus. The pure tone audiogram (PTA) detected some measurable hearing in the right ear at very high intensities. The contralateral left ear showed sloping sensorineural hearing loss. The Weber test, performed with a 512 Hz tuning fork, consistently failed to indicate lateralization, as the patient has reported hearing the tone in the middle of the head. The PTA is shown in Figure 1.

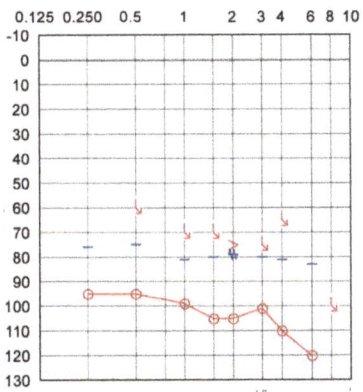 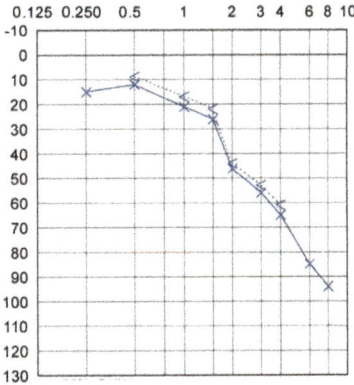

Figure 1. Pure tone audiogram of Patient #1 with right-sided profound hearing loss caused by scarlet fever 72 years ago.

Patient #3: 76-year-old woman who, at the age of 31, underwent a modified radical mastoidectomy for an invasive middle ear cholesteatoma on the right side. As a result of the cholesteatoma and the surgery, the patient had right-sided profound deafness and facial palsy. No recurrence of her cholesteatoma occurred in the following decades. The patient presented to the outpatient department with mastoid cavity problems. The PTA (Figure 2) indicated a sloping hearing loss in the contralateral (left) side with a small air-bone gap after a left-sided tympanoplasty decades ago. The Weber tuning fork test consistently lateralized to the contralateral (left) side, despite the very long UHL duration (45 years).

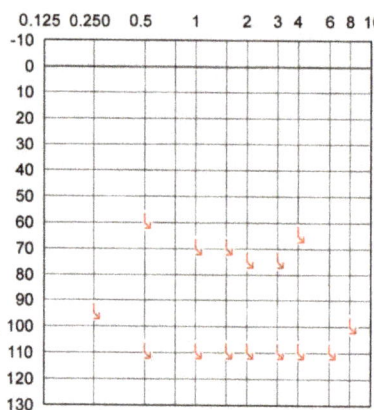 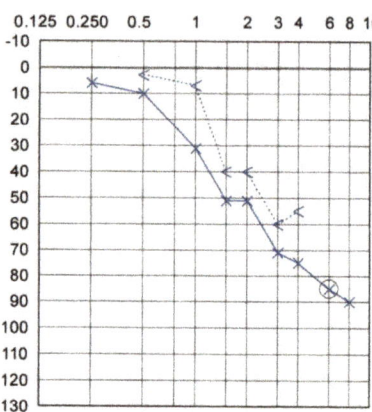

Figure 2. Pure tone audiogram of Patient #3 approximately 45 years after right-sided modified radical mastoidectomy with partial labyrinthectomy for extensive middle ear cholesteatoma.

Patient #4: 54-year-old man who underwent a translabyrinthine surgery for right-sided vestibular schwannoma 17 years ago. Immediately after the surgery, the patient reported a right-sided profound hearing loss (PTA is shown in Figure 3) and facial palsy, both of which have persisted to the present day. The contralateral side retained normal hearing. The magnetic resonance follow-up scans determined no evidence of tumor recurrence, and the Weber test lateralized to the contralateral (left) side.

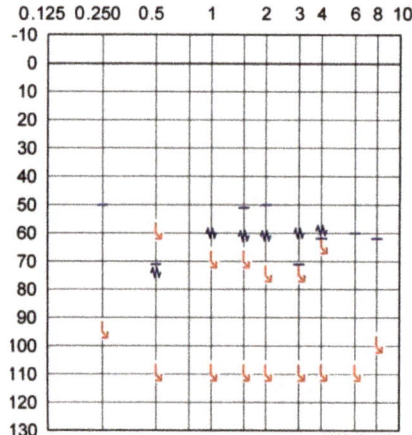 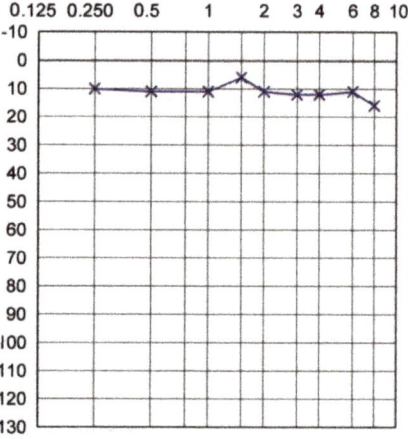

Figure 3. Pure tone audiogram of Patient #4 approximately 17 years after translabyrinthine surgery for right-sided vestibular schwannoma.

Patient #7: 56-year-old woman who suffered from an acute episode of right-sided sudden sensorineural hearing loss (SSNHL) at 46 years. The contralateral side showed normal hearing. Ten years later, the Weber tuning fork test does not lateralize, but instead, it is heard in the middle of the head. The hearing loss and tinnitus did not recover. The patient elected not to undergo cochlear implantation. The PTA is shown in Figure 4.

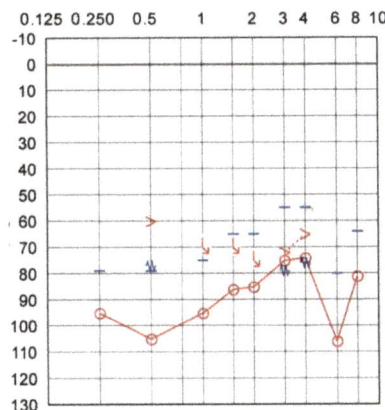 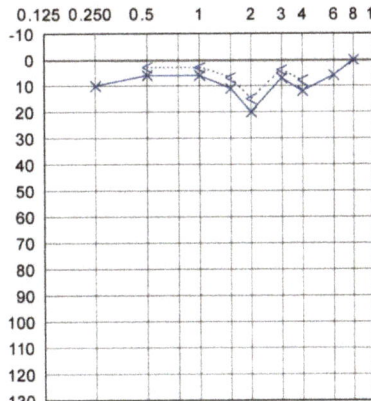

Figure 4. Pure tone audiogram of Patient #7 approximately ten years after right-sided sudden sensorineural hearing loss.

Patient #9: 54-year-old man with profound left-sided sensorineural hearing loss of unknown etiology since birth. The PTA showed contralateral normal hearing (Figure 5). The Weber tuning fork test consistently showed a failure of lateralization.

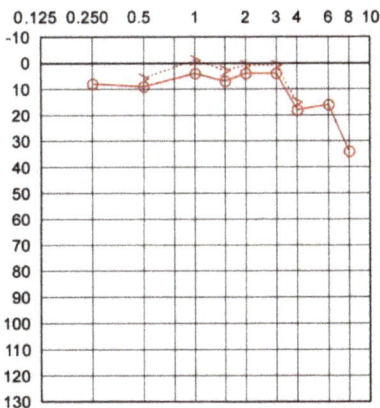 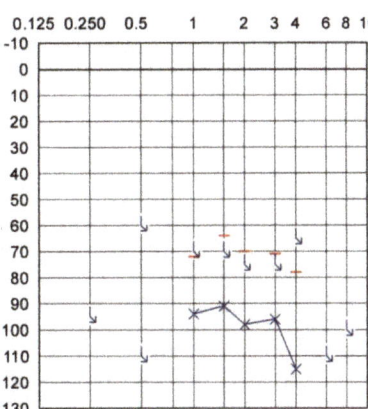

Figure 5. Pure tone audiogram of Patient #9 with left-sided profound hearing loss since birth.

Patient #10 is a 52-year-old man with left-sided Menière's disease for over twenty years. The disease progression had resulted in recurrent vertigo attacks, left-sided sensorineural hearing loss, and tinnitus. After multiple intratympanic gentamicin injections, complete control of the vertigo attacks was reached. However, the intratympanic gentamicin treatment resulted in a left-sided profound UHL for over 18 years. The Weber test lateralized to the contralateral (right) side. The patient was referred to the cochlear implantation unit for auditory rehabilitation. The PTA is shown in Figure 6.

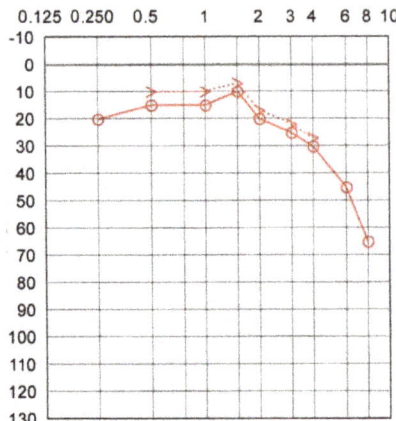 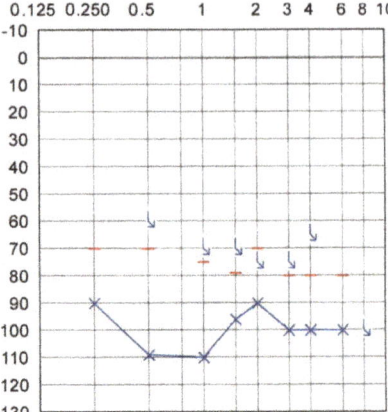

Figure 6. Pure tone audiogram of Patient #10 with left-sided Menière's disease.

4. Discussion

In the present study, we analyzed the results of the Weber test in a small cohort of patients with single-sided deafness (SSD) and asymmetric hearing loss (AHL). The common features shared among all patients in the present study are the unilaterality and long duration of the profound hearing loss, ranging from ten to over seventy years. Despite the anticipated lateralization of the Weber test in the entire cohort, eight of thirteen patients reported the sound heard equally on both sides (no lateralization).

We hypothesize that the longstanding auditory deprivation associated with profound unilateral hearing loss (UHL) could lead to a central adaptation process, contributing to the loss of lateralization of the Weber tuning fork test. This observation appears to apply to both SSD and AHL. It is tempting to speculate that the loss of Weber test lateralization could be attributed to central habituation. Observations from daily otologic practice support such a notion. For instance, patients who underwent successful stapedotomies commonly describe environmental sounds as uncomfortably loud for a short period immediately after the surgery [1]. This observation can be explained by the central adaptation to a low-sound-intensity input from that ear over a long time. Since this discomfort is generally transient, this central adaptation appears to be reversible in those cases of chronic conductive hearing loss [1]. After an acute unilateral vestibular loss, an equivalent central habituation process is also well established [11–13]. It would be interesting to determine whether such an adaptation process in the central auditory system influences the outcome of cochlear implantation in patients with SSD.

The effects of unilateral auditory deprivation on the auditory cortex have been previously studied [14,15]. Children with SSD display neural plastic changes in the auditory cortex, particularly cortical reorganization and interaural preference, which may be reversible after early cochlear implantation [15–18]. Interestingly, auditory cortex maturation continues well into adolescence [19], which may explain the absence of tinnitus and lack of Weber test lateralization observed in patients with postlingual childhood-onset SSD in the present study. These cortical changes may explain the poorer outcome of cochlear implantation in prelingual SSD compared to postlingual SSD [15]. However, animal models of SSD have also shown neuroplastic changes in the subcortical auditory centers [20], making the model even more complex. This complexity renders it challenging to employ specific electrophysiologic or radiological markers as predictors for the outcome of cochlear implantation in patients with longstanding SSD. One potential approach would be to use functional magnetic resonance imaging (fMRI) to evaluate the central reorganization occurring after SSD [21,22]. Based on the current study's findings, we suggest adding the

Weber tuning fork test to the standard test battery to evaluate cochlear implant candidacy in SSD patients.

SSD patients should be counseled about the alternatives to cochlear implantation, including contralateral routing of signals (CROS) or bone conduction devices. While those devices may abolish the head shadow effect, they do not restore binaural hearing [23,24]. In the well-selected motivated SSD patient, cochlear implantation may thus be an attractive treatment option that allows binaural hearing with improved sound localization, tinnitus relief, speech discrimination in noise, and quality of life [25,26]. In a recent randomized controlled trial, cochlear implantation outperformed CROS and bone conduction devices in SSD [26]. However, the auditory outcomes of cochlear implantation in congenital and longstanding SSD still represent a challenge, which was the primary motivation behind the present study, aiming to provide clinical predictors of cochlear implant performance in longstanding SSD.

The lack of reliable electrophysiologic or radiological outcome predictors for cochlear implantation in SSD patients may reflect the incomplete understanding of the neurobiological changes associated with SSD. Indeed, the outcome of cochlear implantation in SSD is variable and depends on several factors, most notably the duration of deafness [27–31]. A long duration of SSD has been associated with poor cochlear implant performance and deficient postoperative speech discrimination [27–31]. As a result, many clinicians do not recommend cochlear implantation in longstanding SSD. However, the outcomes of auditory rehabilitation with cochlear implants vary among SSD patients, precluding a consensus or guideline, since some patients still achieve some degree of benefit even after long durations of deafness [32]. A systematic review of the literature identified a statistically significant negative association between the SSD duration and postoperative speech discrimination [27]. However, the effect size was not clear, thus not allowing for a recommendation on the longest accepted period of SSD for cochlear implant candidacy [27], especially considering the myriad of other confounding factors influencing the outcome. In our own published data on implanted adults with SSD, there was a statistically significant correlation between a longer duration of SSD and poorer postoperative implant performance, with congenital SSD patients having zero speech discrimination in the implanted ear one year after implantation [28,33].

In clinical and experimental studies, the association between tinnitus and SSD has been well established [14]. Chronic subjective tinnitus may be regarded as a central response to peripheral auditory deafferentation [15,34]. Translational audiology experiments with animal models of SSD have demonstrated the lack of tinnitus in congenital SSD [34,35]. This finding has been confirmed by human clinical studies of congenital SSD patients, suggesting that auditory experience is essential for the development of tinnitus [36]. Furthermore, the duration of auditory experience must be sufficiently long for the development of tinnitus [37]. Indeed, Lee and coworkers reported the absence of subjective ipsilesional tinnitus in adult patients with SSD with onset before the age of 20 years [37]. These findings suggest that the lack of tinnitus in SSD may be associated with irreversible neural plastic changes if they persist after the critical point of auditory development in adolescence. As such, the absence of tinnitus in adult patients with childhood-onset SSD may indicate irreversible central changes. Future studies should investigate the potential usefulness of central auditory processing evaluations in detecting those changes. In adult-onset SSD, the role of tinnitus as a predictive factor is less clear. Previous studies have shown that the severity of tinnitus associated with sudden sensorineural hearing loss (SSNHL) decreases with time [38]. Some authors hypothesized that SSD patients with tinnitus might have better auditory outcomes after cochlear implantation than those without tinnitus [39]. In the present study, ipsilesional tinnitus was reported exclusively by patients with adult-onset UHL, which is consistent with the findings of Lee et al. [37]. In the patients with childhood-onset UHL, the absence of tinnitus correlated significantly with the lack of Weber test lateralization. Since our data are only correlative and retrospective, the findings

5. Conclusions

In patients with longstanding SSD referred for cochlear implantation, the poor postimplantation auditory performance can be partially explained by peripheral factors (such as spiral ganglion neurite retraction or neuronal loss). However, a central habituation component is also likely involved, as shown by electrophysiological and brain mapping studies [14,17,40]. It is tempting to hypothesize that the lack of Weber test lateralization could predict this central habituation process, possibly forecasting the auditory performance of implanted SSD patients. Based on this hypothesis, we proposed a novel role for the Weber test as a simple adjunct screening tool before cochlear implantation of SSD patients. If confirmed, this phenomenon may have implications for otologic practice, potentially supporting the decision-making and counseling of patients with longstanding SSD, who seek auditory rehabilitation. Further, more extensive studies are needed to elucidate the relation between the Weber tuning fork test result and the cochlear implant performance in patients with SSD. In addition to clinical research, the reverse translational approach ("bed-to bench") is recommended for further studies to determine the precise cell biology- and neurobiology-based mechanisms of the changes seen in clinical practice.

Author Contributions: Conceptualization, methodology and formal Analysis, M.B.; resources, H.O.; data curation, M.B.; writing—original draft preparation, M.B., S.M.H., S.G., A.J.S. and H.O.; writing—review and editing, M.B., S.M.H., S.G., A.J.S. and H.O.; visualization, M.B.; supervision, A.J.S. and H.O.; project administration, H.O.; funding acquisition, H.O. All authors have read and agreed to the published version of the manuscript.

Funding: This research received no external funding.

Institutional Review Board Statement: The study was approved by the ethics committee of Charité Medical University (approval number EA1/015/21).

Informed Consent Statement: The ethics committee of Charité Medical University has approved the retrospective anonymized analysis of patient data.

Data Availability Statement: Not applicable.

Acknowledgments: The authors thank the audiology staff for their excellent audiometric assessments and collegial collaboration.

Conflicts of Interest: The authors declare no conflict of interest.

References

1. Huizing, E.H. Lateralization of bone conduction into the better ear in conductive deafness. Paradoxical Weber test in unilaterally operated otosclerosis. *Acta Otolaryngol.* **1970**, *69*, 395–401. [CrossRef] [PubMed]
2. Guindi, G.M. Lateralization of the Weber response after stapedectomy. *Br. J. Audiol.* **1981**, *15*, 97–100. [CrossRef] [PubMed]
3. Blakley, B.W.; Siddique, S. A qualitative explanation of the Weber test. *Otolaryngol. Head Neck Surg.* **1999**, *120*, 1–4. [CrossRef]
4. Sichel, J.Y.; Freeman, S.; Sohmer, H. Lateralization during the Weber test: Animal experiments. *Laryngoscope* **2002**, *112*, 542–546. [CrossRef] [PubMed]
5. Scott-Brown, W.G.; Ballantyne, J.; Groves, J. *Scott-Brown's Diseases of the Ear, Nose and Throat: The Ear*; Butterworth: Oxford, UK, 1979.
6. Ghosh, P. Weber-QUO vedis? *Indian J. Otolaryngol. Head Neck Surg.* **1995**, *47*, 140–141. [CrossRef]
7. Goodman, A. Reference zero levels for pure-tone audiometers. *J. Speech Lang. Hear. Res.* **1965**, *7*, 7–16. [CrossRef]
8. Clark, J.G. Uses and abuses of hearing loss classification. *Asha* **1981**, *23*, 493–500.
9. Vincent, C.; Arndt, S.; Firszt, J.B.; Fraysse, B.; Kitterick, P.T.; Papsin, B.C.; Snik, A.; Van de Heyning, P.; Deguine, O.; Marx, M. Identification and evaluation of cochlear implant candidates with asymmetrical hearing loss. *Audiol. Neurootol.* **2015**, *20*, 87–89. [CrossRef]
10. Van de Heyning, P.; Távora-Vieira, D.; Mertens, G.; Van Rompaey, V.; Rajan, G.P.; Müller, J.; Hempel, J.M.; Leander, D.; Polterauer, D.; Marx, M.; et al. Towards a Unified Testing Framework for Single-Sided Deafness Studies: A Consensus Paper. *Audiol. Neurootol.* **2016**, *21*, 391–398. [CrossRef]

11. Curthoys, I.S.; Halmagyi, G.M. Vestibular compensation: A review of the oculomotor, neural, and clinical consequences of unilateral vestibular loss. *J. Vestib. Res. Equilib. Orientat.* **1995**, *5*, 67–107. [CrossRef]
12. Strupp, M.; Arbusow, V.; Maag, K.P.; Gall, C.; Brandt, T. Vestibular exercises improve central vestibulospinal compensation after vestibular neuritis. *Neurology* **1998**, *51*, 838–844. [CrossRef] [PubMed]
13. Dutia, M.B. Mechanisms of vestibular compensation: Recent advances. *Curr. Opin. Otolaryngol. Head Neck Surg.* **2010**, *18*, 420–424. [CrossRef] [PubMed]
14. Gordon, K.; Kral, A. Animal and human studies on developmental monaural hearing loss. *Hear. Res.* **2019**, *380*, 60–74. [CrossRef] [PubMed]
15. Liu, J.; Zhou, M.; He, X.; Wang, N. Single-sided deafness and unilateral auditory deprivation in children: Current challenge of improving sound localization ability. *J. Int. Med. Res.* **2020**, *48*. [CrossRef]
16. Sharma, A.; Glick, H.; Campbell, J.; Torres, J.; Dorman, M.; Zeitler, D.M. Cortical plasticity and reorganization in pediatric single-sided deafness pre- and postcochlear implantation: A case study. *Otol. Neurotol.* **2016**, *37*, e26–e34. [CrossRef]
17. Polonenko, M.J.; Gordon, K.A.; Cushing, S.L.; Papsin, B.C. Cortical organization restored by cochlear implantation in young children with single sided deafness. *Sci. Rep.* **2017**, *7*, 16900. [CrossRef]
18. Lee, H.J.; Smieja, D.; Polonenko, M.J.; Cushing, S.L.; Papsin, B.C.; Gordon, K.A. Consistent and chronic cochlear implant use partially reverses cortical effects of single sided deafness in children. *Sci. Rep.* **2020**, *10*, 21526. [CrossRef]
19. Yamazaki, H.; Easwar, V.; Polonenko, M.J.; Jiwani, S.; Wong, D.D.E.; Papsin, B.C.; Gordon, K.A. Cortical hemispheric asymmetries are present at young ages and further develop into adolescence. *Hum. Brain Mapp.* **2018**, *39*, 941–954. [CrossRef]
20. Kim, S.Y.; Heo, H.; Kim, D.H.; Kim, H.J.; Oh, S.H. Neural plastic changes in the subcortical auditory neural pathway after single-sided deafness in adult mice: A MEMRI study. *Biomed. Res. Int.* **2018**, *2018*, 8624745. [CrossRef]
21. Scheffler, K.; Bilecen, D.; Schmid, N.; Tschopp, K.; Seelig, J. Auditory cortical responses in hearing subjects and unilateral deaf patients as detected by functional magnetic resonance imaging. *Cereb. Cortex* **1998**, *8*, 156–163. [CrossRef]
22. Bilecen, D.; Seifritz, E.; Radü, E.W.; Schmid, N.; Wetzel, S.; Probst, R.; Scheffler, K. Cortical reorganization after acute unilateral hearing loss traced by fMRI. *Neurology* **2000**, *54*, 765–767. [CrossRef] [PubMed]
23. Peters, J.P.; Smit, A.L.; Stegeman, I.; Grolman, W. Review: Bone conduction devices and contralateral routing of sound systems in single-sided deafness. *Laryngoscope* **2015**, *125*, 218–226. [CrossRef]
24. Kitterick, P.T.; Smith, S.N.; Lucas, L. Hearing Instruments for Unilateral Severe-to-Profound Sensorineural Hearing Loss in Adults: A Systematic Review and Meta-Analysis. *Ear Hear* **2016**, *37*, 495–507. [CrossRef] [PubMed]
25. Cabral Junior, F.; Pinna, M.H.; Alves, R.D.; Malerbi, A.F.; Bento, R.F. Cochlear Implantation and Single-sided Deafness: A Systematic Review of the Literature. *Int. Arch. Otorhinolaryngol.* **2016**, *20*, 69–75. [CrossRef] [PubMed]
26. Peters, J.P.M.; van Heteren, J.A.A.; Wendrich, A.W.; van Zanten, G.A.; Grolman, W.; Stokroos, R.J.; Smit, A.L. Short-term outcomes of cochlear implantation for single-sided deafness compared to bone conduction devices and contralateral routing of sound hearing aids-Results of a Randomised controlled trial (CINGLE-trial). *PLoS ONE* **2021**, *16*, e0257447. [CrossRef]
27. Cohen, S.M.; Svirsky, M.A. Duration of unilateral auditory deprivation is associated with reduced speech perception after cochlear implantation: A single-sided deafness study. *Cochlear Implant. Int.* **2019**, *20*, 51–56. [CrossRef]
28. Haussler, S.M.; Kopke, V.; Knopke, S.; Grabel, S.; Olze, H. Multifactorial positive influence of cochlear implantation on patients with single-sided deafness. *Laryngoscope* **2020**, *130*, 500–506. [CrossRef] [PubMed]
29. Kurz, A.; Grubenbecher, M.; Rak, K.; Hagen, R.; Kuhn, H. The impact of etiology and duration of deafness on speech perception outcomes in SSD patients. *Eur. Arch. Oto-Rhino-Laryngol.* **2019**, *276*, 3317–3325. [CrossRef]
30. van Zon, A.; Peters, J.P.; Stegeman, I.; Smit, A.L.; Grolman, W. Cochlear implantation for patients with single-sided deafness or asymmetrical hearing loss: A systematic review of the evidence. *Otol. Neurotol.* **2015**, *36*, 209–219. [CrossRef]
31. Blasco, M.A.; Redleaf, M.I. Cochlear implantation in unilateral sudden deafness improves tinnitus and speech comprehension: Meta-analysis and systematic review. *Otol. Neurotol.* **2014**, *35*, 1426–1432. [CrossRef]
32. Nassiri, A.M.; Wallerius, K.P.; Saoji, A.A.; Neff, B.A.; Driscoll, C.L.W.; Carlson, M.L. Impact of duration of deafness on speech perception in single-sided deafness cochlear implantation in adults. *Otol. Neurotol.* **2022**, *43*, e45–e49. [CrossRef] [PubMed]
33. Haussler, S.M.; Knopke, S.; Dudka, S.; Grabel, S.; Ketterer, M.C.; Battmer, R.D.; Ernst, A.; Olze, H. Improvement in tinnitus distress, health-related quality of life and psychological comorbidities by cochlear implantation in single-sided deaf patients. *HNO* **2020**, *68*, 1–10. [CrossRef] [PubMed]
34. Knipper, M.; van Dijk, P.; Schulze, H.; Mazurek, B.; Krauss, P.; Scheper, V.; Warnecke, A.; Schlee, W.; Schwabe, K.; Singer, W.; et al. The Neural Bases of Tinnitus: Lessons from Deafness and Cochlear Implants. *J. Neurosci.* **2020**, *40*, 7190–7202. [CrossRef]
35. Eggermont, J.J.; Kral, A. Somatic memory and gain increase as preconditions for tinnitus: Insights from congenital deafness. *Hear. Res.* **2016**, *333*, 37–48. [CrossRef] [PubMed]
36. Lee, S.Y.; Nam, D.W.; Koo, J.W.; De Ridder, D.; Vanneste, S.; Song, J.J. No auditory experience, no tinnitus: Lessons from subjects with congenital- and acquired single-sided deafness. *Hear. Res.* **2017**, *354*, 9–15. [CrossRef] [PubMed]
37. Lee, J.M.; Kim, Y.; Ji, J.Y.; Koo, J.W.; Song, J.J. Auditory experience, for a certain duration, is a prerequisite for tinnitus: Lessons from subjects with unilateral tinnitus in the better-hearing ear. *Prog. Brain Res.* **2021**, *260*, 223–233. [CrossRef]
38. Muhlmeier, G.; Baguley, D.; Cox, T.; Suckfull, M.; Meyer, T. Characteristics and spontaneous recovery of tinnitus related to idiopathic sudden sensorineural hearing loss. *Otol. Neurotol.* **2016**, *37*, 634–641. [CrossRef]

39. Liu, Y.W.; Cheng, X.; Chen, B.; Peng, K.; Ishiyama, A.; Fu, Q.J. Effect of tinnitus and duration of deafness on sound localization and speech recognition in noise in patients with single-sided deafness. *Trends Hear.* **2018**, *22*, 1–14. [CrossRef]
40. Kral, A.; Hubka, P.; Heid, S.; Tillein, J. Single-sided deafness leads to unilateral aural preference within an early sensitive period. *Brain* **2013**, *136*, 180–193. [CrossRef]

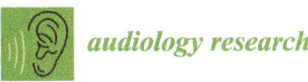

Review

The Otoprotective Effect of Ear Cryotherapy: Systematic Review and Future Perspectives

Dominik Péus [1,2,*], Shaumiya Sellathurai [2,3], Nicolas Newcomb [1,4], Kurt Tschopp [2] and Andreas Radeloff [1]

1. Department of Otorhinolaryngology, University of Oldenburg, 26122 Oldenburg, Germany
2. Department of Otorhinolaryngology, Cantonal Hospital Baselland, 4410 Liestal, Switzerland
3. Department of Biomedicine, University of Basel, 4001 Basel, Switzerland
4. The Software Revolution, Inc., Kirkland, WA 98034, USA
* Correspondence: research.peus@gmail.com; Tel.: +49-441-2360

Abstract: This systematic review investigates ear cooling and cryotherapy in the prevention and treatment of inner ear damage and disease, within the context of animal models and clinical studies. A literature search was carried out in the databases Pubmed and Cochrane Library. Ten studies were identified concerning the otoprotective properties of cryotherapy. Nine of these were rodent in vivo studies (mice, rats, gerbils, guinea pigs). One study involved human subjects and investigated cryotherapy in idiopathic sensorineural hearing loss. The studies were heterogeneous in their goals, methods, and the models used. Disorder models included ischemia and noise damage, ototoxicity (cisplatin and aminoglycoside), and CI-electrode insertion. All ten studies demonstrated significant cryotherapeutic otoprotection for their respective endpoints. No study revealed or expressly investigated otodestructive effects. While limited in number, all of the studies within the scope of the review demonstrated some degree of cryotherapeutic, otoprotective effect. These promising results support the conducting of further work to explore and refine the clinical applicability and impact of cryotherpeutics in otolaryngology.

Keywords: otoprotection; cryotherapy; hypothermia; inner ear

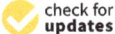

1. Introduction

Pathologic conditions of the inner ear manifest clinically in varying degrees of hearing loss, tinnitus, and dizziness. In some cases, these symptoms severely impair quality of life (QoL) and carry emotional and financial consequences for those affected and their relatives [1,2]. The pathophysiology of many inner ear diseases is not well-known; disorders with a known cause are somewhat better understood. The latter include blast injury, acoustic trauma, or ototoxic hearing loss [3,4]. In contrast, the etiology of disorders such as idiopathic sensorineural hearing loss and acute vestibular neuropathy remain unclear (Schick et al. 2001), although potential suspected causes include autoimmunological processes [5], viral infections [6,7], and vasomotor dysregulation [8]. An improved pathogenetic understanding of these disorders has only sometimes improved therapeutic outcomes.

The two most common therapies for the disorders listed above are steroids and antioxidants; both deliver mixed results in the clinical setting. For example, steroids, despite being a well-established therapy for cisplatin ototoxic hearing loss, do not positively influence outcomes [9]; adverse effects include high blood pressure, blood sugar disorders, and decompensation of psychological comorbidities [10]. Despite substantial testing, the results with antioxidants such as sodium thiosulfate also remain mixed. The 2017 Freyer et al. randomized control trial of oncological diseases in children and young people treated with cisplatin employed an antioxidant containing sodium thiosulfate in the test group, as well as cisplatin [11]. This was regarded as the first effective therapy for cisplatin-induced hearing loss. However, a retrospective analysis demonstrated significantly worse

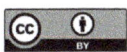

QoL in the test group with advanced tumor disease [12]. As a result, a potential reduction by the antioxidant of cisplatin's anti-cancer activity cannot be ruled out. At present, known otoprotective therapies are both limited in their availability and applicability, and demonstrate questionable efficacy.

In the search for better otoprotective therapies, clinicians and researchers are evaluating novel therapeutic modes. To this end, the otoprotective effect of cryotherapy (otoprotective hypothermia, OH) has been investigated since the 1980s, and a number of in vivo studies have been published. It is somewhat surprising that local cooling in otorhinolaryngology (with a few exceptions) has not been studied more actively, considering thermal manipulation of the inner ear is an established clinical routine in the diagnosis of the vestibular organ, and the broad protective effects of cryotherapy are included in intensive care medicine and oncology (prevention e.g., scalp hair loss during chemotherapy) daily routine [13–15].

In this review we seek to elucidate the following key topics: (i) the current state of application and understanding of cooling of the inner ear; (ii) the protective effect of cooling on hearing; (iii) the pros and cons of cryotherapy in human otolaryngology disorders; and (iv) potential methods of administering cryotherapy.

2. Methods

A literature search was conducted between 1 September and 30 September, and again between 1 December 2021 and 31 January 2022, according to PRISMA guidelines [16]. Search parameters included (a) condition (e.g., hearing loss, deafness, blast injury, tinnitus, hair cell loss) and (b) intervention (e.g., hypothermia, cryotherapy, cooling). The terms and Boolean combinations were adapted for the database searches in Pubmed and the Cochrane Library. Figure 1 demonstrates the search outcomes as a PRISMA flow diagram. Literature cited within the included studies was also reviewed. No restrictions were placed on the date of publication. Studies from the search sample set described above were included in the review if they explored effects of cooling on the inner ear.

For this review, two review authors (DP and SS) independently searched and identified eligible studies and trials based on the following characteristics: study population (clinical studies, or in vivo studies) and study intervention (clinical study recruiting probands with an inner ear disease receiving or not receiving cryotherapy; inner ear model of a cochlear damage with or without cryotherapy).

The review authors screened titles and abstracts to identify potentially relevant citations. The full text of the article was retrieved and reviewed when the title and abstract screening were ambiguous in their relevance. The review authors independently assessed the eligibility of the studies, by filling out eligibility forms designed in accordance with the review study inclusion criteria.

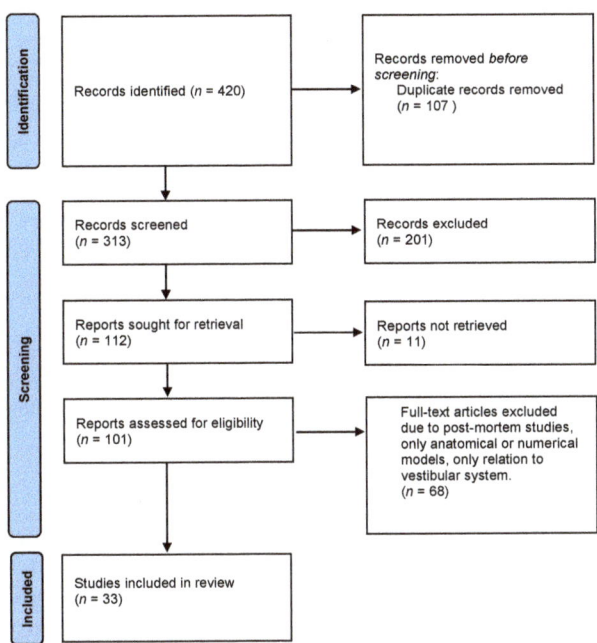

Figure 1. Flow chart of the study selection procedure.

3. Results

The studies included in the review were heterogeneous in their objectives, the animal models used, how cold was applied, and measurement methods. A total of 33 studies were identified investigating the impact of cooling on the inner ear. However, only 10 studies of the 33 investigated the otoprotective potential of cryotherapy in the ear. The remaining 23 studies were more heterogenous and focused on fundamental research.

3.1. Cooling Effects on Compound Action Potential

Fifteen of the twenty-three studies investigating the impact of cooling on the cochlea, without reference to otoprotection, used animal models. Five of these in vivo studies investigated the impact of cooling on compound action potentials (CAP) [17–21]. Brown et al. measured CAP in guinea pigs with whole-body hypothermia and used 1-ms rise–fall time to evoke the CAP. Small changes were observed when cooling to between 37 °C and 34 °C. With further cooling, amplitude, waveform, threshold, and latency changed greatly and mostly reversibly. The amplitude decrease in the high frequencies was explained by a selective decrease in the sensitivity of units tuned to higher frequencies. However, the increase in the latency of units was independent of their characteristic frequency. The authors presume that this could be explained by the fact that the conduction velocity of myelinated nerves decreases linearly with the decrease in temperature.

3.2. Cooling Effects on Endocochlear Potential and Single nerve Fibers

Cooling has been shown to reduce the endocochlear potential (EP) in the base of the guinea pig cochlea, from 86 mV to 73.2 mV on average, after 2 h of cooling, reaching a rectal temperature 29 °C [22]. Two studies investigated the impact of cooling on the endocochlear potential (EP), as facilitated by the stria vascularis [20,22]. Single auditory nerve fiber recordings were used by two studies, which suggested that mechanical properties were more changed in the base of the cochlea then in the apex. This further supports the validity of CAP and EP cooling findings [23,24].

3.3. Cooling Effects on Otoacoustic Emissions

Temperature dependence of distortion product (DPOAE) and transient evoked otoacoustic emissions (TEOAE) were found in at least three studies [25–27]. No changes were observable between 37 °C and 33–34 °C, but DPOAE and TEOAE were significantly, but reversibly, suppressed at temperatures below the lower range.

3.4. Other In Vivo Studies

Few studies used non-electrophysiological measures. Miller et al. published several papers using laser Doppler flowmtry to measure the cochlear blood flow in guinea pigs. They exposed the bone of the basal turn of the cochlea to a cryoprobe. This induced a reduction of the cochlear blood flow for cryoprobe temperatures of −40 °C compared to 0 and −10 °C [28,29].

The studies listed above prove that in vivo cooling leads to reversible changes of the different components of the inner ear, with a tendency to most strongly affect the base of the cochlea. However, investigations upon the cooling application itself were not systematic or closely comparable across studies.

3.5. Comparison of Cooling Administration

Only two in vivo studies were identified comparing different application methods of cooling. Smith et al. 2007 used a rat model and placed a temperature micro-probe in the basal flexion of the cochlea. Water irrigation over the external ear canal (EEC) was compared with an opened bulla approach [30]. EEC irrigation with water cooled to 14 °C and 11 °C decreased cochlear temperature on average by 1.1 °C and 1.6 °C, respectively. Bulla irrigation with water cooled to 14 °C and 11° decreased cochlear temperature on average by 3.3 °C and 4.1 °C, respectively. Stanford et al. 2020 compared EEC irrigation and a thermoelectrically cooled metal ear bar in a guinea pig model. The ear bar needed to be cooled to temperatures 7 °C lower than the EEC irrigation temperature, to achieve similar cooling effects [31]. These two studies demonstrated that cooling applied locally over the external ear canal leads to temperature changes within the inner ear in vivo. In contrast, most other in vivo studies used whole-body hypothermia. Localized cooling methods are more interesting, clinically, than whole-body hypothermia, due to the more practical route to clinical application.

3.6. Cooling-Induced Otoacoustic and Temperature Changes in Human Studies

Temperature measurements in the tissues, cells, or fluid compartments of the inner ear in living human subjects are lacking. As a result, surrogate measurements such as otoacoustic emissions were used in five studies. During cardiac surgeries whole-body hypothermia was applied. It was shown that the TEOAE and DPOAE response is dependent on the body core temperature [32–36].

Two human studies measured induced temperature change on the surface of the bony labyrinth [37,38]. Kleinfeld and Dahl measured temperature variations at the lateral bony canal during 11 ear surgeries (posterior tympanotomies). Cooling was applied by filling up the external ear canal with about 2 ml 20 °C tempered or 0 °C tempered water. The mean temperature decrease was 0.8 °C and 1.2 °C within 70 s. However, the administration of only 2 mL cooling fluid is not likely to be sufficient to cool down the inner ear. What remains unclear is what temperature change can practically be provoked in living human subjects with EEC cooling or neck cooling, nor are the methods described that explain how temperature changes should be measured within the inner ear in living human subjects without the need for surgery.

3.7. Evidence of Cryotherapy for Prevention and Therapy

Ten studies investigating the otoprotective effects of cooling were identified. Of these, nine were in vivo studies with rodents; one was a clinical study of hearing loss in human patients. Table 1 summarizes the included papers, sorted by investigated effect and localization of cooling.

Table 1. Study characteristics.

Results	Whole-Body	Ectopic, Cervical	Invasive, Promontory	Ear Canal
Increase of the cochlear ischaemic tolerance	Takeda et al. 2008 (gerbils) Watanabe et al. 2001 (gerbils) Hyodo et al. 2001 (gerbils)			
Decrease of noise damage	Henry et Chole 1984 (mice, gerbils) Henry 2003 (mice)			
Increasing the residual hearing after CI	Balkany et al. 2005 (rats)		Tamames et al. 2016 (rats)	
Increased rate of cured patients after sudden idopathic hearing loss		Hato et al. 2010 (human)		
Decrease of cisplatin ototoxicity				Spankovich et al. 2016 Stanford et al. 2020 (guinea pigs)

Decrease in cisplatin ototoxicity: Two studies by the Spankovich group demonstrated protection of hair cell activity in guinea pigs under the application of non-invasive cooling of the outer ear canal [31,39]. Spankovich et al. irrigated the outer ear canal for 20 min with 30 °C water, 2 h before administering a single dose of cisplatin (12 mg/kg, i.p.). The same research group refined their methods for a later 2020 study and used a more accurate cisplatin dosing regimen of one application per week (4 mg/kg, i.p.) for 3 weeks, which cumulatively reached dose equivalence with Spankovich et al. (12 mg/kg) [31]. The results of Spankovich and Stanford did not significantly differ. Cisplatin exposure over time resulted in minimal, insignificant ABR and DPOAE measurement threshold shifts for the control and intervention groups. After the second cisplatin dose, there was a significant threshold shift in the control group, a small, nonsignificant threshold shift in the intervention group, and no significant difference between the two groups. After the third dose, a significantly greater threshold shift was shown in the control group compared to the cooled group. In addition, hair cell loss in the cochlear basal region was significantly reduced for the intervention group [31]. In short, pre-emptive cryotherapy was successfully demonstrated to protect hearing and hair cells from repeated cisplatin exposure.

Cranial cooling in the treatment of idiopathic hearing loss: While the etiology of idiopathic sensorineural hearing loss has not been clarified, many forms of therapy have been tested. Hato et al. conducted a multi-center study [40], motivated by the otoprotective effect of hypothermia observed in the ischemia model of Watanbe et al. [41]. The patients in Hato et al.'s study hypothermic group (N = 86) were admitted and treated with a cooled water pillow for 48 h, in addition to standard treatment for 7 days, which was 60 mg prednisolone for days 1–3 and reduced doses days 4–7, and 60 mg of Adenosine Triphosphate (ATP) and 150 mg of methylcobalamin over 7 days. The water pillow was cooled to 15 °C and was changed 4–5 times per day. The patients used the water pillow for the first 48 h after admission, with restricted activity. The control patients received only the medications. No adverse effects of the cooling pillow therapy were observed. At 6 months, there was no observable statistical case-matched analysis difference in patients aged 60 years or older. The below 60 years of age subgroup showed a statistically significantly higher recovery rate, i.e., 71.4% vs. 46.5% in the control group [40]. Complete recovery was defined as hearing level recovered within 20 dB at five frequencies (0.5, 1, 2, 4, and 8 kHz) or hearing level recovered to that of the contralateral, unaffected ear.

Increasing cochlear ischemia tolerance as a model for idiopathic hearing loss: Some animal studies model idiopathic hearing loss by disconnecting blood supply to the cochlea. These studies showed that mild full-body hypothermia (32 °C) reduced and usually also prevented hearing loss, as measured in terms of brain stem audiometry and immunohistochemistry (number of intact hair cells) when compared to the normothermic group [41–44].

Reduction of the destructive effect of acoustic trauma: Henry et al. demonstrated the protective effects of cryotherapy within the context of acoustic trauma in mice and gerbils [45]. They exposed mice and gerbils of different ages to noise (5 min, 8–16 kHz octave band, 115 dB SPL). They then measured the cochlear action potential, before and after noise exposure, at 4 days. The damage was quantified as a threshold shift in dB. The average permanent threshold shift (PTS) was 37.2 dB in young mice in the normothermic group. In the mild hypothermic group (30 °C) the average PTS was 26 dB. An electron micrograph of the apical, mid, and basal parts of the cochlea was taken. The authors asserted that the physiological findings support CAP measurements, without providing a further quantitative analysis.

Increasing residual hearing after cochlear implantation (CI): Balkany et al. conducted a rat-based animal study demonstrating improved residual hearing after CI in animals treated with systemic hypothermia (34 °C) [46]. They investigated the effect of mild hypothermia on hearing loss due to electrode insertion trauma in normal hearing rats. Electrode insertion leads to cochlear damage, which is clinically relevant in functional deaf patients with residual hearing, i.e., at low frequencies. ABR threshold shift was substantially reduced in the hypothermia group (-4.2 dB SPL) vs. the normothermia group (-15.9 dB SPL). Similarly, Tamames et al. demonstrated significant otoprotection in a hypothermia group, quantified as reduced ABR shift and improved hair cell count [47]. The main difference between the Tamames and Balkany studies was in the application of cooling. Balkany et al. used mild whole-body hypothermia; Tamames et al. explored cold application to the cochlear promontory via a rod-like device.

4. Discussion

The research, conclusions, and ultimately cryotherapy's clinical usefulness as a therapeutic approach remain a fragmented picture. In vivo study results are promising, and positive physiological effects in the inner ear were observed, but this evidence pertains mostly to full-body hypothermia, which is impracticable for use in clinical studies, and probably impractical in most clinical settings. The reviewed works applied thermal energy eclectically, so while the methods do not strongly corroborate one another, the results are still generally promising. Furthermore, the varied studies show multiple clinically interesting hypothermic impacts on the inner ear. Cryotherapy applications variously increased ischemic tolerance, reduced cisplatin ototoxicity, and reduced both acoustic trauma and residual hearing loss as caused by the CI electrodes. Nevertheless, little is known about the mechanisms that take place within the inner ear in hypothermic conditions. Taken together, these studies and measurements demonstrated that hypothermia has an effect, and frequently enough a beneficial effect; however, it remains unclear how that effect unfolds, and corroborating studies would be advisable to prioritize the form of application and verify preliminary results in the areas where doing so would have the greatest impact; i.e., QoL impacting clinical areas where other therapies are lacking or where otological damage is particularly severe.

Most of the in vivo studies had a relatively simple design and relied upon a combination of hypothermic exposure in combination with different potentially hearing-harming conditions and electrophysiological measurement, e.g., a hair-cell count. These captured measurable changes, but were not generally sufficiently precise in application, to ascertain what methods of application affect electrophysiological change most effectively, or why. Several studies investigated electrophysiological changes in CAP, CP, and OAE, and thereby demonstrated hypothermic effects at the basal part of the cochlea. CAP amplitude, waveform, threshold, and latency changed significantly, and mostly reversibly, below 32–34 °C (body core temperature) [17]. In the case of the cisplatin-model the main mechanism is, in all likelihood, reduced blood flow and, therefore, a reduced uptake of ototoxic substances, e.g., cisplatin [48]. Additional mechanisms of action might include slowed metabolism, reduced oxidative stress, and the involvement of cold shock proteins [49]. Higher metabolic and mechanical activity might explain the higher susceptibility of high-frequency areas vs. low-frequency areas of the cochlea.

It is worthwhile to further explore the theoretical physiology of cooling. Cooling reduces the blood flow of the stria vascularis and, therefore, impacts the endocochlear potential, but it is unclear whether the vasoconstriction (and therefore a reduced blood flow) on the level of the cochlea is responsible for some of the reported therapeutically promising observations, or if further systemic changes within the body (e.g., reduced cardiac output following whole-body hypothermia) are responsible for the effect [22,29].

Furthermore, not all the physiological phenomena are explained by processes in the organ of Corti or the stria vascularis, because increased CAP latency was also observed. This implies a hypothermia-associated process in the first neuron. This simply reinforces the lack of clarity as to whether slowed metabolism or reduced perfusion, or perhaps neither or both, are responsible for neural changes. Future research regarding physiological changes of the inner ear should use models that more precisely localize cooling at the ear, avoiding full body hypothermia, to differentiate better local cooling effects and exclude more general processes. Furthermore, methods should be applied that support the investigation of hypothermia-associated changes on an intracellular level with a differentiation between the different cell types, to further uncover the precise mechanism by which therapeutic effects are being achieved (or to hint at potentially undesirable side-effects).

There are a number of otologic diseases currently lacking reliable therapy options, and which are potential targets for cryotherapy. Within this context, at present, the state of the available literature implies that there is no consensus related to the prioritization of which pathological condition or conditions might be best suited for study. In terms of the most applicable therapeutic methods, only neck-applied cooling pad otoprotective hypothermia studies have been conducted in humans, and these were entirely limited to idiopathic hearing loss [40]. It is questionable whether idiopathic hearing loss is the most relevant application for cryotherapy in otology disorders, and whether neck cooling is a sufficient therapy for the disorder. Idiopathic sudden hearing loss is difficult to investigate because of the unclear, possibly diverse, etiologies and the resultant variable time frames at which patients should be enrolled in a study. A further obstacle is the high spontaneous remission rates. The single study exploring otoprotection in humans by Hato et al. is promising but is insufficient for actionable, clinical conclusions to be drawn, related to the protective or therapeutic potential of cryotherapy in otorhinolaryngology.

Cisplatin-induced hearing loss might be a reasonable candidate for translational research with cryotherapy, because the etiology is well understood [12]. Further arguments for prioritizing cryotherapy for cisplatin-induced hearing loss, include the fact that the ototoxic agent is known (which improves quantifiable evaluation, due to the dose-dependency of the ototoxicity). Studies could be schedulable to consistent time frames in the ototoxic progression (time of drug administration), and a study group is clearly available as control, as cisplatin is generally ototoxic in healthy-hearing patients.

Other disorders, which have not been explored in this work, and for which studies were not discovered in our review (and presumably do not exist), but which also are potential cryotherapy candidates, include vestibular neuritis, zoster oticus, and middle ear infection with inner ear involvement. A characterization of the prevalence of these ailments, the scope of otological damage, and a review of the therapies generally available for these conditions would be useful in identifying which of these might be most suitable for exploring the usefulness of cryotherapy in care. These diseases were, of course, outside the scope of this review, because, to date, cryotherapy has not been attempted (or at least not attempted and published). A reasonable cryotherapeutic trial protocol, may be an accessible and efficient path to new QoL improvements for these disorders.

Besides prioritizing the best disease targets for future study, the cryotherapeutic protocol (mentioned above) seems to be a prime target for optimization and standardization. In short, the method of cooling that is best for otoprotective therapy has not yet been established. Disease targeting is inextricably connected to the question of how cryotherapy is applied to the human body. Hato et al. used neck cooling to ectopically cool. However, the approach of neck cooling is not new and is under debate for brain protection, e.g., out-of-hospital reanimations. Neck with full-head cooling was used in healthy volunteers and intensive care unit patients [50–52], demonstrating a temperature drop at the tympanic membrane of around 0.8–1.5 °C, with a significant reflexive increase in blood pressure. Sole use of neck cooling is probably not ideal for future cryotherapy trials, because of its potential inefficiency and side-effects.

Ear canal cooling seems practicable as a therapeutic vehicle. Cooling takes place close to the target organ (the inner ear) and would not obviously cause severe or unpredictable effects. Two studies were identified in which induced temperature change was measured in humans, and where the EEC was inundated with water [37,38]. Spankovich et. al. used EEC cryotherapy to reduce cisplatin toxicity in guinea pigs [31,39]. Notably, no human otoprotective study with an EEC approach seems to have been conducted yet. However, the procedure is basically known, is used, and is safe. Simultaneous bilateral application of caloric stimulation is a known and proven method. Studies have investigated its *diagnostic* value for the testing of the vestibular system and also central vestibular lesions [53–55]. Bilateral *therapeutic* cryotherapy should, therefore, also be feasible.

With regards to long-term cooling methods, due to the lack of a suitable long-term cooling device, there is no data available to conclude whether longer cooling durations of, for example, an hour or longer, are acceptable. Long-term cooling, in any case, would not seem to be a practical implementation.

Besides duration, the degree of cooling that is appropriate has also not yet been established. Mild local hypothermia may prove tolerable but insufficient to achieve effective otoprotection. This too requires exploration, though general cryotherapeutic studies should be useful to establish safe parameters for such explorations.

Through a focus upon cryotherapy for ototherapeutic purposes, it should be possible to arrive at reasonably standardized methods, which can better help to elucidate the otoprotective mechanisms and applications relevant to further develop new, useful, and cost-effective therapeutic applications for ototoxic disease.

5. Conclusions

Otoprotective cryotherapy is a therapeutic approach that has been proven by various in vivo studies. Although the studies were quite heterogeneous in terms of methodology and objectives, they demonstrate protective effects and carry clinical potential. Future in vivo studies on otoprotective cryotherapy should investigate molecular–genetic, metabolic, and cellular mechanisms, in addition to verifying otoprotective key outcomes (i.e., ABR and hair cell count). A better understanding of these mechanisms in all cells of the inner ear, including hair cells and support cells, as well as the stria vascularis, would help to guide future development of therapeutic methods, regardless of whether these are cryotherapy-oriented or not. Data on the tolerability and safety of bilateral, simultaneous cold application would be desirable, as such "soft" factors determine the acceptance and, thus, success in patients. Significant research effort is required to empirically provide grounds for clinical targets, methods, and recommendations. We recommend beginning such research in the diseases best understood, and then leveraging such useful principles as can be proven to drive further scientific and clinical progress.

Author Contributions: Conceptualization, D.P. and A.R.; methodology, D.P., S.S. and A.R.; validation, D.P. and S.S.; formal analysis, D.P. and S.S.; writing—original draft preparation, D.P., S.S., N.N., K.T. and A.R.; writing—review and editing, D.P., S.S., N.N., K.T. and A.R.; supervision, D.P. and A.R.; funding acquisition, D.P. All authors have read and agreed to the published version of the manuscript.

Funding: This study was supported by the Research Fund 2020 3MS1052 of the University of Basel.

Institutional Review Board Statement: Not applicable.

Informed Consent Statement: Not applicable.

Data Availability Statement: Not applicable.

Conflicts of Interest: The authors declare no conflict of interest.

References

1. Dixon, P.R.; Feeny, D.; Tomlinson, G.; Cushing, S.; Chen, J.M.; Krahn, M.D. Health-Related Quality of Life Changes Associated With Hearing Loss. *JAMA Otolaryngol. Neck Surg.* **2020**, *146*, 630–638. [CrossRef]
2. Mohr, P.E.; Feldman, J.J.; Dunbar, J.L.; McConkey-Robbins, A.; Niparko, J.K.; Rittenhouse, R.K.; Skinner, M.W. The societal costs of severe to profound hearing loss in the United States. *Int. J. Technol. Assess. Health Care* **2000**, *16*, 1120–1135. [CrossRef]
3. Kellerhals, B. Pathogenesis of inner ear lesions in acute acoustic trauma. *Acta. Otolaryngol.* **1972**, *73*, 249–253. [CrossRef]
4. Szczepek, A.J. Ototoxicity: Old and New Foes. In *Advances in Clinical Audiology*; Hatzopoulos, S., Ed.; InTech: London, UK, 2017.
5. Cadoni, G.; Fetoni, A.R.; Agostino, S.; Santis, A.D.; Manna, R.; Ottaviani, F.; Paludetti, G. Autoimmunity in sudden sensorineural hearing loss: Possible role of anti-endothelial cell autoantibodies. *Acta Otolaryngol. Suppl.* **2002**, *122*, 30–33. [CrossRef]
6. Merchant, S.N.; Durand, M.L.; Adams, J.C. Sudden deafness: Is it viral? *ORL J. Otorhinolaryngol. Relat. Spec.* **2008**, *70*, 52–60. [CrossRef]
7. Stokroos, R.J.; Albers, F.W. The etiology of idiopathic sudden sensorineural hearing loss. A review of the literature. *Acta Otorhinolaryngol. Belg.* **1996**, *50*, 69–76.
8. Ballesteros, F.; Tassiesm, D.; Reverter, J.C.; Alobid, I.; Bernal-Sprekelsen, M. Idiopathic sudden sensorineural hearing loss: Classic cardiovascular and new genetic risk factors. *Audiol. Neurootol.* **2012**, *17*, 400–408. [CrossRef]
9. Rybak, L.P.; Mukherjea, D.; Jajoo, S.; Ramkumar, V. Cisplatin ototoxicity and protection: Clinical and experimental studies. *Tohoku J. Exp. Med.* **2009**, *219*, 177–186. [CrossRef]
10. Wei, B.P.C.; Stathopoulos, D.; O'Leary, S. Steroids for idiopathic sudden sensorineural hearing loss. *Cochrane Database Syst. Rev.* **2013**, *7*, CD003998. [CrossRef]
11. Freyer, D.R.; Chen, L.; Krailo, M.D.; Knight, K.; Villaluna, D.; Bliss, B.; Pollock, B.H.; Ramdas, J.; Lange, B.; Van Hoff, D.; et al. Effects of sodium thiosulfate versus observation on development of cisplatin-induced hearing loss in children with cancer (ACCL0431): A multicentre, randomised, controlled, open-label, phase 3 trial. *Lancet Oncol.* **2017**, *18*, 63–74. [CrossRef]
12. Minasian, L.M.; Frazier, A.L.; Sung, L.; O'Mara, A.; Kelaghan, J.; Chang, K.W.; Krailo, M.; Pollock, B.H.; Reaman, G.; Freyer, D.R. Prevention of cisplatin-induced hearing loss in children: Informing the design of future clinical trials. *Cancer Med.* **2018**, *7*, 2951–2959. [CrossRef]
13. Grevelman, E.G.; Breed, W.P.M. Prevention of chemotherapy-induced hair loss by scalp cooling. *Ann. Oncol.* **2005**, *16*, 352–358. [CrossRef]
14. Monzack, E.L.; May, L.A.; Roy, S.; Gale, J.E.; Cunningham, L.L. Live imaging the phagocytic activity of inner ear supporting cells in response to hair cell death. *Cell Death Differ.* **2015**, *22*, 1995–2005. [CrossRef]
15. Royl, G.; Füchtemeier, M.; Leithner, C.; Megow, D.; Offenhauser, N.; Steinbrink, J.; Kohl-Bareis, M.; Dirnagl, U.; Lindauer, U. Hypothermia effects on neurovascular coupling and cerebral metabolic rate of oxygen. *Neuroimage* **2008**, *40*, 1523–1532. [CrossRef]
16. Page, M.J.; McKenzie, J.E.; Bossuyt, P.M.; Boutron, I.; Hoffmann, T.C.; Mulrow, C.D.; Shamseer, L.; Tetzlaff, J.M.; Akl, E.A.; Brennan, S.E.; et al. The PRISMA 2020 statement: An updated guideline for reporting systematic reviews. *BMJ* **2021**, *372*, n71. [CrossRef]
17. Brown, M.C.; Smith, D.I.; Nuttall, A.L. The temperature dependency of neural and hair cell responses evoked by high frequencies. *J. Acoust. Soc. Am.* **1983**, *73*, 1662–1670. [CrossRef]
18. Fernandez, C.; Singh, H.; Perlmann, H. Effect of short-term hypothermia on cochlear responses. *Acta Otolaryngol.* **1958**, *49*, 189–205. [CrossRef]
19. Harrison, J.B. Temperature Effects on Responses in the Auditory System of the Little Brown Bat Myotis l. lucifugus. *Physiol. Zool.* **1965**, *38*, 34–48. [CrossRef]
20. Ohlemiller, K.K.; Siegel, J.H. The effects of moderate cooling on gross cochlear potentials in the gerbil: Basal and apical differences. *Hear Res.* **1992**, *63*, 79–89. [CrossRef]
21. Shore, S.E.; Nuttall, A.L. The effects of cochlear hypothermia on compound action potential tuning. *J. Acoust. Soc. Am.* **1985**, *77*, 590–598. [CrossRef]
22. Konishi, T.; Salt, A.N.; Hamrick, P.E. Effects of hypothermia on ionic movement in the guinea pig cochlea. *Hear Res.* **1981**, *4*, 265–278. [CrossRef]
23. Gummer, A.W.; Klinke, R. Influence of temperature on tuning of primary-like units in the guinea pig cochlear nucleus. *Hear Res.* **1983**, *12*, 367–380. [CrossRef]
24. Ohlemiller, K.K.; Siegel, J.H. Cochlear basal and apical differences reflected in the effects of cooling on responses of single auditory nerve fibers. *Hear Res.* **1994**, *80*, 174–190. [CrossRef]
25. Khvoles, R.; Freeman, S.; Sohmer, H. Effect of temperature on the transient evoked and distortion product otoacoustic emissions in rats. *Audiol. Neurootol.* **1998**, *3*, 349–360. [CrossRef] [PubMed]

26. Meenderink, S.W.; van Dijk, P. Temperature Dependence of Anuran Distortion Product Otoacoustic Emissions. *J. Assoc. Res. Otolaryngol.* **2006**, *7*, 246–252. [CrossRef]
27. Noyes, W.; McCaffrey, T.; Fabry, D.; Robinette, M.; Suman, V. Effect of temperature elevation on rabbit cochlear function as measured by distortion-product otoacoustic emissions. *Otolaryngol. Head Neck Surg.* **1996**, *115*, 548–552. [CrossRef]
28. Miller, J.M.; Goodwin, P.C.; Marks, N.J. Inner ear blood flow measured with a laser Doppler system. *Arch. Otolaryngol.* **1984**, *110*, 305–308. [CrossRef]
29. Miller, J.M.; Marks, N.J.; Goodwin, P.C. Laser Doppler measurements of cochlear blood flow. *Hear Res.* **1983**, *11*, 385–394. [CrossRef]
30. Smith, L.P.; Eshraghi, A.A.; Whitley, D.E.; van de Water, T.R.; Balkany, T.J. Induction of localized cochlear hypothermia. *Acta Otolaryngol.* **2007**, *127*, 228–233. [CrossRef]
31. Stanford, J.K.; Morgan, D.S.; Bosworth, N.A.; Proctor, G.; Chen, T.; Palmer, T.T.; Thapa, P.; Walters, B.J.; Vetter, D.E.; Black, R.D.; et al. Cool OtOprotective Ear Lumen (COOL) Therapy for Cisplatin-induced Hearing Loss. *Otol. Neurotol.* **2021**, *42*, 466–474. [CrossRef]
32. Borin, A.; Cruz, O.L.M. Study of distortion-product otoacoustic emissions during hypothermia in humans. *Braz. J. Otorhinolaryngol.* **2008**, *74*, 401–409. [CrossRef]
33. El Ganzoury, M.M.; Kamel, T.B.; Khalil, L.H.; Seliem, A.M. Cochlear Dysfunction in Children following Cardiac Bypass Surgery. *ISRN Pediatr.* **2012**, *2012*, 1–6. [CrossRef]
34. Seifert, E.; Lamprecht-Dinnesen, A.; Asfour, B.; Rotering, H.; Bone, H.G.; Scheld, H.H. The influence of body temperature on transient evoked otoacoustic emissions. *Br. J. Audiol.* **1998**, *32*, 387–398. [CrossRef] [PubMed]
35. Seifert, E.; Brand, K.; van de Flierdt, K.; Hahn, M.; Riebandt, M.; Lamprecht-Dinnesen, A. The influence of hypothermia on outer hair cells of the cochlea and its efferents. *Br. J. Audiol.* **2001**, *35*, 87–98. [CrossRef] [PubMed]
36. Veuillet, E.; Gartner, M.; Champsaur, G.; Neidecker, J.; Collet, L. Effects of hypothermia on cochlear micromechanical properties in humans. *J. Neurol. Sci.* **1997**, *145*, 69–76. [CrossRef]
37. Kleinfeldt, D.; Dahl, D. Temperaturmessungen am Menschlichen Bogengang Nach Thermischer Reizung. *Acta Otolaryngol.* **1969**, *68*, 411–419. [CrossRef]
38. Schmaltz, G. The physical phenomena occurring in the semicircular canals during rotatory and thermic stimulation. *Proc. R. Soc. Med.* **1931**, *25*, 359–381.
39. Spankovich, C.; Lobarinas, E.; Ding, D.; Salvi, R.; Le Prell, C.G. Assessment of thermal treatment via irrigation of external ear to reduce cisplatin-induced hearing loss. *Hear Res.* **2016**, *332*, 55–60. [CrossRef]
40. Hato, N.; Hyodo, J.; Takeda, S.; Takagi, D.; Okada, M.; Hakuba, N.; Gyo, K. Local hypothermia in the treatment of idiopathic sudden sensorineural hearing loss. *Auris Nasus Larynx* **2010**, *37*, 626–630. [CrossRef]
41. Watanabe, F.; Koga, K.; Hakuba, N.; Gyo, K. Hypothermia prevents hearing loss and progressive hair cell loss after transient cochlear ischemia in gerbils. *Neuroscience* **2001**, *102*, 639–645. [CrossRef]
42. Hyodo, J.; Hakuba, N.; Koga, K.; Watanabe, F.; Shudou, M.; Taniguchi, M.; Gyo, K. Hypothermia reduces glutamate efflux in perilymph following transient cochlear ischemia. *Neuroreport* **2001**, *12*, 1983–1987. [CrossRef]
43. Takeda, S.; Hakuba, N.; Yoshida, T.; Fujita, K.; Hato, N.; Hata, R.; Hyodo, J.; Gyo, K. Postischemic mild hypothermia alleviates hearing loss because of transient ischemia. *Neuroreport* **2008**, *19*, 1325–1328. [CrossRef] [PubMed]
44. Takeda, S.; Hata, R.; Cao, F.; Yoshida, T.; Hakuba, N.; Hato, N.; Gyo, K. Ischemic tolerance in the cochlea. *Neurosci. Lett.* **2009**, *462*, 263–266. [CrossRef] [PubMed]
45. Henry, K.R.; Chole, R.A. Hypothermia protects the cochlea from noise damage. *Hear Res.* **1984**, *16*, 225–230. [CrossRef]
46. Balkany, T.J.; Eshraghi, A.A.; Jiao, H.; Polak, M.; Mou, C.; Dietrich, D.W.; Van De Water, T.R. Mild hypothermia protects auditory function during cochlear implant surgery. *Laryngoscope* **2005**, *115*, 1543–1547. [CrossRef]
47. Tamames, I.; King, C.; Bas, E.; Dietrich, W.D.; Telischi, F.; Rajguru, S.M. A cool approach to reducing electrode-induced trauma: Localized therapeutic hypothermia conserves residual hearing in cochlear implantation. *Hear Res.* **2016**, *339*, 32–39. [CrossRef]
48. Miller, J.M.; Ren, T.Y.; Nuttall, A.L. Studies of inner ear blood flow in animals and human beings. *Otolaryngol. Head Neck Surg.* **1995**, *112*, 101–113. [CrossRef]
49. Spankovich, C.; Walters, B.J. Mild Therapeutic Hypothermia and Putative Mechanisms of Hair Cell Survival in the Cochlea. *Antioxid Redox Signal* **2021**, *36*, 1203–1214. [CrossRef]
50. Koehn, J.; Kollmar, R.; Cimpianu, C.L.; Kallmünzer, B.; Moeller, S.; Schwab, S.; Hilz, M.J. Head and neck cooling decreases tympanic and skin temperature, but significantly increases blood pressure. *Stroke* **2012**, *43*, 2142–2148. [CrossRef]
51. Koehn, J.; Wang, R.; de Rojas Leal, C.; Kallmünzer, B.; Winder, K.; Köhrmann, M.; Kollmar, R.; Schwab, S.; Hilz, M.J. Neck cooling induces blood pressure increase and peripheral vasoconstriction in healthy persons. *Neurol. Sci.* **2020**, *41*, 2521–2529. [CrossRef]
52. Poli, S.; Purrucker, J.; Priglinger, M.; Diedler, J.; Sykora, M.; Popp, E.; Steiner, T.; Veltkamp, R.; Bösel, J.; Rupp, A.; et al. Induction of cooling with a passive head and neck cooling device: Effects on brain temperature after stroke. *Stroke* **2013**, *44*, 708–713. [CrossRef]

53. Furman, J.M.; Wall, C.; Kamerer, D.B. Alternate and simultaneous binaural bithermal caloric testing: A comparison. *Ann. Otol. Rhinol. Laryngol.* **1988**, *97*, 359–364. [CrossRef] [PubMed]
54. Hoffman, R.A.; Brookler, K.H.; Baker, A.H. The accuracy of the simultaneous binaural bithermal test in the diagnosis of acoustic neuroma. *Laryngoscope* **1979**, *89*, 1046–1052. [CrossRef] [PubMed]
55. Sataloff, R.T.; Pavlick, M.L.; McCaffrey, J.D.; Davis, J.M.; Stewart, S.M. Simultaneous binaural bithermal caloric testing: Clinical value. *Ear Nose Throat J.* **2017**, *96*, 29–31. [PubMed]

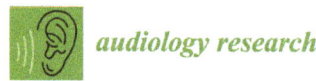

Obituary

In Memoriam: David Mark Baguley

Don McFerran [1,*] and Laurence McKenna [2]

[1] British Tinnitus Association, Woodseats Close, Sheffield S8 0TB, UK
[2] Department of Clinical Psychology, Royal National ENT and Eastman Dental Hospitals, University College Hospital, 47–49 Huntley St, London WC1E 6DG, UK
* Correspondence: donmcferran@aol.com

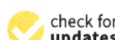

Citation: McFerran, D.; McKenna, L. In Memoriam: David Mark Baguley. *Audiol. Res.* **2022**, *12*, 585–588. https://doi.org/10.3390/audiolres12060057

Academic Editor: Giacinto Asprella Libonati

Received: 19 October 2022
Accepted: 19 October 2022
Published: 24 October 2022

Publisher's Note: MDPI stays neutral with regard to jurisdictional claims in published maps and institutional affiliations.

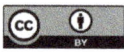

Copyright: © 2022 by the authors. Licensee MDPI, Basel, Switzerland. This article is an open access article distributed under the terms and conditions of the Creative Commons Attribution (CC BY) license (https://creativecommons.org/licenses/by/4.0/).

Reverend Professor David (Dave) Mark Baguley, audiologist, hearing scientist, tinnitus clinician, educator, and Church of England priest, died suddenly and unexpectedly in Nottingham, UK on 11 June 2022, at the age of 61 (Figure 1). Dave was preceded in death by his mother Sheila. He is survived by his wife Bridget; their children Sam, Naomi and Luke; his father, Philip and his brothers Peter and Richard.

He was born on the 18 March 1961 in Manchester, UK. The family relocated to Ipswich, Suffolk but Dave never lost his Mancunian roots, and remained a fervent lifelong supporter both of Manchester City soccer team and of Manchester Indie Music. After attending Northgate Grammar School for Boys in Ipswich (now Northgate High School) he returned to study at Manchester University where he was awarded a BSc (Hons) in Psychology in 1983, and subsequently an MSc in Clinical Audiology in 1985.

After university, his first job was as Scientific Officer at the Medical Research Council (MRC) Institute of Hearing Research in Cardiff, Wales. After eight months in this post, he moved to Addenbrookes Hospital in Cambridge UK, working for the National Health Service (NHS) as an Audiological Scientist. Four years later he became Head of Audiology and was later awarded Consultant status. He remained at Addenbrookes Hospital for over 30 years and the Audiology Department grew under his stewardship to achieve international renown. Latterly, he added Head of Hearing Implants to his job description and became Clinical Lead for the local neonatal hearing screening service. As part of the process of developing the Audiology Department, he instigated Cambridge's first dedicated Tinnitus Clinic in 1987.

To support his growing managerial responsibilities, he studied for an MBA which was awarded with Distinction by the Open University in 1994. His academic career was also blossoming and by this stage his medical writing was in full flow. He was contributing to the peer-reviewed medical press at a prodigious rate and ultimately wrote more than 220 scientific articles. The main thrust of his initial research and writing concerned vestibular schwannomas but by the late 1990s his research direction had shifted, and the publication emphasis became tinnitus and hyperacusis. Although he wrote many erudite papers, he seemed most fond of some of his quirkier publications. Finding a niche that no-one else had considered gave him great pleasure and resulted in one paper about positive experiences of tinnitus, another about the international vocabulary of tinnitus and a book chapter on tinnitus and hyperacusis in literature, film, and music. This offbeat approach spilled into his presentations which were often scattered with tinnitus references from literature and the arts: even Tintin featuring in one of his talks! While continuing to work full-time, he undertook a PhD on the physiological mechanisms of tinnitus in patients with vestibular schwannoma. This degree was awarded by Cambridge University in 2005.

Throughout his tenure at Addenbrookes, Dave developed what was to become a lifelong passion for teaching, and this extended not only to audiology staff but also to both the homegrown medical trainees passing through the ENT Department and the international research fellows who were attached to the hospital's skull base team. This ability to cross boundaries into other clinical and research disciplines was one of Dave's strongest points: he was equally comfortable talking to a young audiologist, a senior ENT surgeon, a representative of big pharma, a psychologist or the head of a large university department. This skill, combined with an encyclopaedic knowledge of tinnitus and hyperacusis research, ensured that he became the go-to person for people wanting advice on new research topics or novel tinnitus treatments. It also ensured that he became an unusual entity: an audiologist who was comfortable speaking at big ENT events. He presented several times at the Otology section of the Royal Society of Medicine and the UK's leading ENT conference, the British Academic Conference in Otolaryngology (BACO).

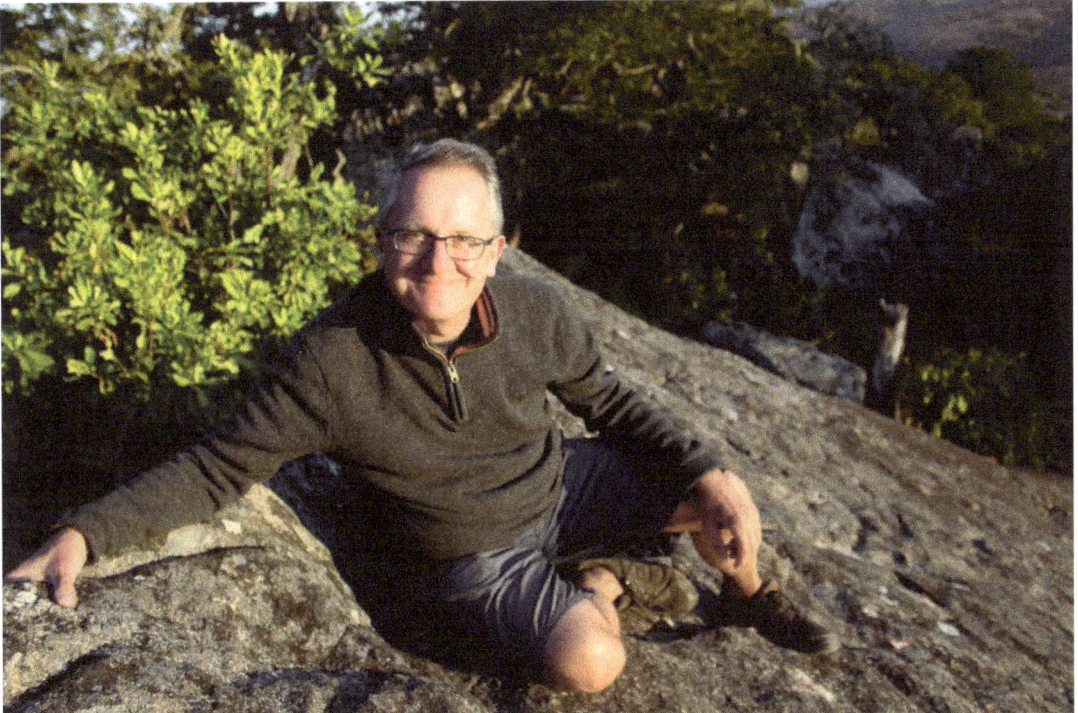

Figure 1. Photo of Professor David (Dave) Mark Baguley.

The ability to move seamlessly between clinical, research and industry settings made his opinion almost indispensable in matters of translational research: nearly all the recent trials of potential tinnitus drugs or therapeutic devices sought Dave's views prior to commencement. He was passionate in his view that tinnitus should be approached as a team effort and that only by adopting a multidisciplinary approach could we hope to move forward.

Dave cared deeply about his work, and this is one of the factors that helped to make him such an extraordinary teacher. On hearing of Dave's death one colleague said: "I can remember so clearly everything he taught me. It was impossible to attend a lecture he gave without coming away with your mind changed or challenged about something in a way that usually led to a more compassionate outlook or understanding. And somehow, he did it without making you wrong for having thought about it differently." Dave taught on many courses, including the long-running European Tinnitus Course. He was always happy to have detailed and careful conversations about the content of his lectures, over coffee, lunch, even breakfast the following morning, or indeed, later via email. He was available to all. In the words of another colleague: "In the big scheme of things, no one would ever know me really, I'm just an everyday audiologist yet Dave always included me and reached out to share information or respond to questions as if I were important. He made me feel important." His care was also very evident in his clinical work. At times this made him irascible if he felt others were not putting in the same effort, but these occasional outbursts were usually short lived, and he was adept at defusing such situations with a sprinkling of wit and charm.

In 2007, Dave took a brief sabbatical from Cambridge and for four months undertook the role of Raine/Phonak Visiting Professor at the University of Western Australia, Perth, Australia. A year after his return he was offered a UK University Chair and became Visiting Professor at Anglia Ruskin University in Cambridge and Chelmsford in 2009.

In addition to journal articles, Dave wrote countless book chapters and was editor for books on tinnitus, hearing loss and hyperacusis. He co-authored two tinnitus books: one textbook for professionals, Tinnitus, a multidisciplinary approach; one self-help book for people with tinnitus and hyperacusis, Living with tinnitus and hyperacusis. Both books were well received and are in their second editions.

Dave contributed to many organisations and committees at local, national, and international level. He was a regular speaker at the local tinnitus support group in Cambridge. He was Chair of the British Society of Audiology, 2009–2011, and was editor of their periodical, the British Journal of Audiology (now the International Journal of Audiology) from 1995–2000. His vision helped to create the British Academy of Audiology. Dave joined the Editorial Board of the journal ENT News in 2008 and was instrumental in expanding the remit of the journal to include audiology, resulting in a name change to ENT & Audiology News. He was a member and subsequently Chair of the Professional Adviser's Committee of the British Tinnitus Association and served as its President from 2015 to 2019. He sat on a Department of Health committee developing tinnitus commissioning guidelines. Dave was involved in the formation of the international committee of the American Academy of Audiology and served as co-chair for three years.

Dave was the recipient of numerous prizes and awards, including the Marie and Jack Shapiro Research Prize of the British Tinnitus Association on no less than five occasions, the TS Littler Research Prize from the British Society of Audiology (1994), the International Award of the American Academy of Audiology (2006), the Golden Lobe Award from the Association of Independent Hearing Healthcare Practitioners (2016), and the Norman Gamble Research Prize from the Royal Society of Medicine (2018).

In 2016 Dave decided on a career change and relocated to the University of Nottingham, taking up the position of Professor of Hearing Sciences within the School of Medicine's Division of Clinical Neuroscience. He was Deputy Lead of the Hearing Theme in the Nottingham National Institute for Health and Care Research (NIHR) Biomedical Research Centre. Projects that he was involved with included investigation of hearing loss and tinnitus following platinum-based chemotherapy, development of a hearing bioresource, and a clinical trial on new adult hearing aid users, funded by the Health Technology Assessment Programme.

From his 20s onwards Dave developed a deep Christian faith and in characteristic fashion he chose to take a very active role: in 2011 he received a Diploma in Pastoral Theology from Anglia Ruskin University and was ordained Deacon in the Church of England. In 2012 he was ordained at Ely Cathedral as Priest in the Church of England. When the family relocated to Nottingham, Dave's wife Bridget took on the Ministry of St Martin's Church, Sherwood and Dave became Associate Minister.

Music featured highly in Dave's life. He had eclectic tastes that encompassed everything from Van Morrison to Lee Scratch Perry to The Broken Family Band. However, undoubtedly his greatest admiration was for the Manchester band Joy Division and its rebirth as New Order. He was a keen attender of live music events, particularly the annual Cherry Hinton Folk Festival. Dave was an enthusiastic musician himself, playing rhythm guitar and it was a great source of pride to him that his children had embraced his joy of music.

One might be forgiven for thinking that there would be little room for anything else in Dave's life, but he had many other interests: voracious reader, talented cook, hill walker, family man and above all, he loved to sit and chat, preferably over a pint or two of real ale.

Author Contributions: Conceptualization, D.M.; Investigation, D.M. and L.M.; writing—original draft preparation, D.M. and L.M.; writing—review and editing, D.M. and L.M.; supervision, project administration, D.M. All authors have read and agreed to the published version of the manuscript.

Funding: This research received no external funding.

Institutional Review Board Statement: Not applicable.

Informed Consent Statement: Not applicable.

Data Availability Statement: Not applicable.

Acknowledgments: We would like to thank Marc Fagelson and Glynnis Tidball for their constructive comments and advice on an earlier version of this manuscript.

Conflicts of Interest: The authors declare no conflict of interest.

MDPI
St. Alban-Anlage 66
4052 Basel
Switzerland
www.mdpi.com

Audiology Research Editorial Office
E-mail: audiolres@mdpi.com
www.mdpi.com/journal/audiolres

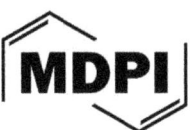

Disclaimer/Publisher's Note: The statements, opinions and data contained in all publications are solely those of the individual author(s) and contributor(s) and not of MDPI and/or the editor(s). MDPI and/or the editor(s) disclaim responsibility for any injury to people or property resulting from any ideas, methods, instructions or products referred to in the content.

www.ingramcontent.com/pod-product-compliance
Lightning Source LLC
LaVergne TN
LVHW070554100526
838202LV00012B/466